Operation Caregivers:
#LifewithDementia

By

Alexandra Allred, M.S.

Cover design created by T.M. Franklin

All photographs are courtesy of the author, Michelle and Diana Powe.

The Next Chapter Publishing Paperback Edition Published 2017

Library of Congress Cataloging-in-Publication Data has been applied for.

ISBN: 978-0-692-96170-4

Table of Contents

Dedication

One might suspect this work would be dedicated to my parents and, at first glance, one would be right. Throughout the process of writing this book and the progression of our parents' decline, however, I've come to understand whom this special note of praise needs to be given.

To caregivers around the world—specifically those who care for, love, and honor parents who are not their own—thank you. What amazing people you are.

Acknowledgments

To Londa, with her contagious laughter, Maria, Christeen, Kamal, Merle, Yaya, Cheryl, Rose, Mari Grace, and Shandell, thank you for bringing our father back to us.

To Maria L., Linda, and Pamela, thank you for being Mom's friend when she's at her most unfriendly. Lilian and Georgia, thank you! To Jeanette, thank you for always having our back. And Norma, thank you for your sweet patience with our father.

It is impossible to name everyone at Isle at Watercrest, but please know we are indebted to your kindness and professionalism.

Beyond this particular band of beautiful people, we also want to thank *all* caregivers, whether you work in facilities or make special trips to the home. You provide a kind of love and patience that is beyond measure. You are a gift to humanity.

To you, the reader. Thank you. Thank you for reading about this very important topic. Please note that in honor of my father, the book was formatted in similar manner to his many military field manuals.

Thank you, DJ Gann, for editing this most challenging story and for the brilliant idea for the book cover. Thank you, T.M. Franklin, for making the cover a reality.

Thank you, Uncle Stephen, for being our advisor, our go-to guy, our guru. Thank you, Aunt Diana, for playing back-up QB and master of all things 'research.' Finally, a HUGE 'thanks – xxoo!' to family, friends, and Facebook buddies who spurred this project on. Your love and support are what got us through…

Preface

It's 2 am. Do you know where your parents are?
We're not entirely sure where—oh, there they are…moving a couch!

This journey first began while our parents were still living outside Washington, D.C., and my sister, Michelle, and I noticed our mother was suddenly unavailable…like, all the time! Every time either of us called, our father always answered the phone. After fifty years of giving his best Joe Friday impression—*Just the facts, ma'am*—and saying very little, it was odd hearing a chatterbox with his voice on the other end of the line. Particularly since he's pretty much deaf and hardly ever paid attention to what we said when he did hear it, which made for wildly inappropriate responses.

As weeks turned into months, our conversations became increasingly frustrating. So much so that either Michelle or I eventually gave into our frustrations and yelled, "Well, okay, then. Can I just please speak to Mom?"

A few times we managed to get her on the phone, but more often than not, she was simply unreachable, busy, or performing some task requiring her full and immediate attention and needed to—but never did—call us back.

Given our upbringing, when we hit our limit, we were prepared. We launched a full-on assault, aptly named *Operation Relocation*. It was time to get Mom and Daddy moved to Texas. It just made sense. By our reasoning, they could see their grandchildren more often, the cost of living was much lower in Texas than the District of Columbia area, and we were available to help with anything needing help.

Mom was dead set against any such move, but we remained steadfast—thank goodness—and at long last, our dad agreed.

We had no idea what we were getting into.

I went 'round and 'round before I typed the first word of this book. Sure, I'd written nonfiction before, but this was such a serious topic. It wouldn't have my trademark humor and intrigue—or would it? And if it did, how much should I share? Where was the fine line between our parents' privacy and full disclosure to readers—still strangers—about information we wished someone had shared with us before this emotional, physical, and mental roller coaster began? And if we shared, were we telling stories out of turn or making the diseases of Alzheimer's and dementia more relatable? And if it was okay, should I go into detail—the depression, lost dreams, massive debt, strained relations, addiction, not to mention skirting concerns for national security? After all, if I was going to tell it, shouldn't all the gory bits be shown?

For all my doubts and insecurity, Facebook told me what I needed to know.

I began posting—mostly to keep a stranglehold on my own sanity and humor. I created my own *LifewithDementia* hashtag and wrote about my father's strange new infatuation with my mother's T-shirts, their late-night wandering, and my mother's insistence that her husband was having an affair. Titles like *How Bingo Really Works in a Memory-Care Facility, They Call My Father Jason Bourne: The Man Who Can Escape a Locked-in Facility Moving at a Snail's Pace*, and *What Not to Do at 2 am in a Locked-in Memory-care Unit* were my personal therapy.

The response was both cathartic and telling.

I picked up over five hundred new friends on Facebook who left a variety of comments.

> "I know this is so frustrating for you, but you have GOT to write a book or make this into a reality show!"
> "When the movie comes out, I want front-row tickets."
> "I want to laugh, I want to cry. Thank you for sharing your parents with everyone."

I received hundreds of private messages thanking me for offering the brutal truth about life in memory care and *#LifewithDementia*, but it was standing in line at my local bank, when the teller made a passing comment as she took care of business, that sealed the deal.

"You post stuff about your parents on Facebook, don't you? One of our other patrons was telling us about it."

The resulting conversation was the day I knew this story was needed.

While there is no doubt ours is an unusual story in the details, the end result is ours is no different than anyone else fighting and surviving Alzheimer's and dementia. It is cruel. It is unfair. Either one of these diseases brings confusion, chaos, and extreme sadness with it, but the two together are an especially vicious double whammy.

The flip side of that coin is that they can also bring laughter, tremendous clarity, and a greater appreciation for the things you had and have.

For us, that coin flip came within twenty-four hours of the day we "lost" our parents, so to speak. As we delved into the world of impenetrable passwords, encoded emails, incomprehensible medical diagnoses, and discovered the depletion of more than fifty thousand dollars in the months leading up to that horrible day we were forced to come to terms with unresolved family issues.

Let it be known that the lunacy under which we currently live is not representative of who our parents once were, and so this is not simply the story of one couple succumbing but evidence of how entire communities are impacted by these diseases. This is a book about four people—Marc and Karen Powe, pre-dementia, and Marc and Karen Powe, the victims. It is also, hopefully, the start of a discussion about the very things we don't like talking about—growing up and getting old.

Getting old is hard. Growing up is even harder.

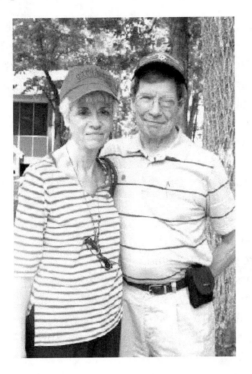

Marc and Karen Powe

FACEBOOK POST: May 2016

For those who live w/ and love someone with Alzheimer's, conversations can be taxing. Try having it in stereo—two parents! But THREE? Holy cow. Today went to visit parents but was joined with another resident, Sylvia (who is 50% extremely sweet, 50% volatile). The conversation began because I brought my dad a hamburger and ALLLLL I was saying was, "You can eat it now or save it for later." Here we go:

Father: It appears …(loses train of thought)

Mom: What's in that box? Is it cake?

Sylvia: Cake? Oh, I want some.

Alex: No, I brought a burger for Daddy. I'm sorry. I could bring—

Sylvia: Oh, no. He can't have that.

Father: It appears…

Sylvia: No! I cannot have that.

Mother: [to me] There she goes again. She's—

Father: …that the doors are closed. Oh! [sees burger]

Sylvia: No! He can't have that. We are having cake tonight.

Father: [hands burger to me]

Alex: [trying to ignore other two] You don't want a burger?

Father: On the west side…

Alex: You could have this now if you want.

Sylvia: He can't have that cake. No! No! No!

Mother: …not that anyone listens to me. What do I know?

Sylvia: The cake is for later. Later. We will sing.

Mother: I had my hat but now they took it and we have to have cake now.

Sylvia: There is no cake.

Mother: I was not talking to you!

Alex: Mom. She's just…

Mother: I know what she is doing. She wants to tell everyone what to do. And now I have to find my hat!

Father: This is my hat, I suppose [now clearly worried about the hat situation]

Mother: …but they took it like they take everything else

Sylvia: That doesn't LOOK like cake!

Mother: Who has cake?

Alex: There is no cake. No cake. I brought this burger for Daddy but…

Sylvia: No! He cannot have that.

I gave up and said, "You know what? I think I'll put this cake in your room, Daddy!" and started to walk off.

Sylvia called after me. "Where are you taking that cake?"

Mom: You have cake?

NOOOOO. No cake! None. Zippo. There is no cake. Never was.

She followed me all the way to the room talking about cakes and hats and a horse saddle. Gawd. I walked her back to the cafeteria and I'll be…but they were serving cake. I can't. I just can't.

Oh, but I can.

Chapter One

FACEBOOK POST: *August, 2016*

> *Alex: [to caregiver] Well, the one thing I know for certain in this lifetime is that my*
> *mother would never use foul language!*
> *Mom: [voice raised, in another room] Those bitches can't keep their hands off of my*
> *husband!*
> *Alex: But then, I really don't know much so...*

Dad had punched Kimberly...in the face.

It was not representative of the man we knew. The man we grew up with was not at all violent

and would never lay hands on a woman. The very idea was mortifying, on so many levels. Yet, it

was true. What was worse, we adored Kimberly. She's one of the good ones.

In fact, that was my first reaction—*Why* Kimberly*? Man! If he's going to punch someone, why*

not Attila?

Okay, that's not her real name, but by the time we landed in this joint, Attila, aka the Hun, aka I-

get-paid-to-do-this-job-but-don't-see-why-that-means-I-should-actually-get-out-of-my-seat-to-

work, aka #AddictedToMyCellphone, seemed determined to step forward as a shining example

of what's wrong in our senior healthcare system. And Attila wasn't alone.

Let me backtrack a moment. To clarify, Michelle and I didn't go from *Operation Relocation* to

stuffing our parents in a facility overnight. No, sir! What started as a simple idea—get Mom and

Daddy moved closer to us—became a long, drawn out, physically draining, complicated

emotional steroid of mind-boggling torture as we came to terms with the undeniable fact that we

had no choice but to place them into some sort of care facility What's worse? Everyone suffered

as we continued trying to be the obedient, dutiful daughters we were raised to be before we came

to the difficult decision that we were beyond our capabilities and understanding of handling what

was going on mentally and physically with our parents.

Your parents take care of you when you're a child, and as they grow older, when it's time, it's your turn to take care of them. That's what being a good child/son/daughter means. That's what we're taught, right?

So…how did we end up here? With Attila and her cronies roaming the memory-care facility with ease and our dad popping wonderful nurses, like Kimberly, in the face?

One facility at a time, my friend.

At this point in my parents' story, we'd interacted with quite a few caregivers who were anything but caring…or giving, for that matter. Counting the hospital and a rehab center, our father had been in six different facilities within ten months.

While he has never been an easy man to deal with, he's never done anything to deserve being left on his own, disoriented and overmedicated into compliant complacency, to fall repeatedly as he tries to maneuver around this foreign (to him) environment until the moment someone finally gets around to checking on him only to discover he's covered in his own fecal matter. He's never done anything to deserve being forced into a cold shower, naked and afraid, then scrubbed and berated until someone else deems him clean again. He has done nothing to deserve being victimized by repeated thefts or locked in a room because it's easier than actually dealing with him as a living, breathing being.

Kimberly understood that from the start. She was the real deal—a true caregiver—which was why learning that our father hit her was worse than the act of violence itself.

Punching Attila in the face? *Tempting*. But Kimberly? *No way!*

"I just don't want them to think this is who he is," Michelle said as I sat, nodding in numb agreement.

We had the conversation concerning our father's new personality many times over before we got to this stage of the dementia game. Those discussions triggered our decision to surround Daddy with his awards and medals and work his heroic efforts for this great nation into any and every conversation we were a part of…so the nursing-care aids could better understand this great man who also happened to be our father. He wasn't some mean old man. He wasn't the belligerent old codger they saw before them.

Marc Powe was one of the most highly decorated military intelligence officers in United States history. This was the same guy responsible for getting a photograph of the undercarriage of a Soviet tank that the Pentagon had been drooling over for three decades. The same guy who gathered intelligence on Yasser Arafat and walked the streets of Baghdad, calmly reporting the goings-on, while mortars fell around him. Our dad was one of only a handful of guys who, when the American Embassy was set ablaze in 1977 Moscow, refused to leave his post as suspected KGB operatives posed as firefighters tried to break into top-secret files, and then Daddy topped the night off by saving the American flag from burning. The guy who was taken hostage by the Kuwaiti government after discovering the Soviets transporting heavy artillery and weapons into the Middle East in the 80s.

Yeah. *That* guy! That's the guy who punched Kimberly.

Gawd, Daddy! Why?

While I contemplated emailing the owner of the facility to make sure Kimberly was okay and offer yet another heartfelt apology, Michelle was already launching into full-scale wooing mode via *Operation Love Kimberly*.

From the outset of this journey, one of our main strategies has been ensuring the staff of every facility liked us, which also meant liking our mom, and as increasingly difficult as he was making it, our father. After all, if we were entrusting our father's health and happiness, such as it was, to these caregivers, shouldn't we get to know them? And vice versa?

We doggedly strove to take part in pleasant—albeit sometimes awkward and forced—conversations with Attila and the other not-so-great caregivers and made it our business to know aspects of their personal lives so we could relate, share, and build some sort of bond wherever possible. And when Daddy went on a tear, we made sure we brought goodies—pastries, Starbucks, colas, you name it—as peace offerings on our father's behalf.

Despite promises of *quality care* touted by the almost five-thousand-dollar-a-month facility and very clear job descriptions on the part of the staff receiving their part of that charge with every paycheck, the harsh reality was many of these uninspired women (and a few men) were far too comfortable sitting around staring at their cell phones.

Rather than recognizing that they—of their own accord—had decided to get into the business of senior care, taken an oath, and made a commitment to give proper attention to their clients/patients in exchange for monies received, it had become evident these givers of questionable care were accustomed to watching over mostly sedentary and docile Alzheimer's patients and were none too happy about having to stand and walk. They had no desire to give anything extra to a retired military colonel who, after severe head trauma, thought he was a prisoner of war.

In other words, they did not want to actually have to work for their dollar.

The reality is, by the year 2030, it is projected there will be approximately seventy-two million people over the age of sixty-five in the United States. As cases of dementia, Alzheimer's, Parkinson's, not to mention basic aging, rise, the need for professionals trained in the art of attending to the elderly is going to be massive and knowing Attila and her cronies are who we have out there "caring" for seniors is upsetting.

Very upsetting.

The events that occurred next were the basis for this book, so perhaps, in hindsight, we owe a backhanded thanks to these un-professionals because we hope to shine a light on a very flawed system in play for our senior citizens.

On six separate occasions, the nineteen-dollar-an-hour sitter from the outside-care facility walked off the job during the wee hours of the night because they, too, were into the very easy gig of watching old people sleep and, even better, watching Netflix and their social media accounts from their cell phones, and were not prepared for the very active colonel.

He has always been that way.

Working and travelling with Colonel Marc B. Powe meant no leisure time, no breaks, no lunches. When he was working, he never stopped, rarely slept, and barely ate. He was a relentless pit bull.

Our father's reputation was widely known, even among his Pentagon peers who knew him as *the White Knight*. Daddy earned the nickname for his brutally honest answers, complete devotion to his nation and flag, and dogged determination to complete whatever mission he was assigned, personal safety be damned. In fact, he made a few enemies in the CIA after the White Knight snuck in under the radar and gathered intel out from under special agents' noses more times than the agency cared to admit.

The truth was, at one time, he was the very best at what he did and *couldn't* be stopped, which was why his mind tricking him into replaying those events over and over at each new facility he entered was doubly hard to take.

One of the nicest things to come out of this entire situation has been the number of retired military personnel—from majors all the way up the military ladder to generals—willing to share their stories about either the character of the man we knew as our father or his White Knight notoriety. Turns out, once upon a time, our father led more soldiers than we ever knew into battle, through covert operative missions, and in the classroom. Time and again we heard how his "was one of the most brilliant minds" of our times.

Their tales were unexpected gifts for my sister and me. As much as Daddy may not appreciate the scuttlebutt, with every story, we began to understand just how many crashes (planes and cars) our dad had survived, how many guns had been aimed at him, and how many verbal threats had been made against his life. It wasn't until we heard the tales that we realized just how inside the spy world our father really had been.

How do you not feel overwhelming pride after that? Our father was James Bond *and* Batman rolled into one hell of a White Knight!

Our father never volunteered mission details with us. He was immensely humble and, for the sake of national security, quiet. Our dad, the White Knight, did not approve of Chris Kyle's tell-all-and-then-some book about his life in the military, and Daddy cringed at the idea of insiders talking about who shot Osama bin Laden. True military intelligence officers did not tell tales—true or then-some.

Oddly, had Daddy not fallen, I doubt we would have ever known these stories.

Only a few times have we been able to discover something about our father on our own.

Such was the case in 2002.

Following the attacks on American soil, September 11, 2001, when General Powell went to Baghdad, I recall standing in my kitchen, watching CNN, when—just for a moment—I spotted a figure on the back side of a pillar before he ducked out of sight again. *I swear, that looked like Daddy!* Sure enough, after further review, there was the Colonel—the White Knight—standing vigil at a press conference when he realized a camera was aimed in his direction. In the very next frame, he was gone.

He was covert all the way and probably hated that even an instant of a second was ever caught on film.

I taunted him about it for years afterward while he repeatedly denied knowing what I was talking about.

He denied being anywhere. He never outright lied, but he was skilled in the ways of artfully dodging mission of anything, and there's no better example of that than the New York Times Best Sellers book *The Billion Dollar Spy* by David Hoffman.

As I flipped through pictures covering the time frame we lived in Moscow, Russia, I came across a photo that got my full attention. "Daddy, there's a picture of you in this book!"

He looked up. "Oh, I don't think so," he said, in the most casual way.

In the past, our dad had served as an anonymous source for two very large news agencies and a very, *very* well-known reporter (one which we are truly not at liberty to reveal). To have his photograph in a book this popular, however, was indeed unusual.

Hmm. "That's you!" I flipped the book around, pointing at the photo.

He scowled. "If you say so."

It's him.

Learning details about those covert operations, however, also gave us insight. The motivation for what everyone, including us, had assumed were eccentricities of dementia began clicking into place—our elderly father, now dealing with the aftereffects of a significant head injury, was still playing the role of the White Knight as he astonished nurses and aids by dismantling restraints, a wheelchair, and even part of his bed.

"Was he some kind of engineer?" everyone asked.

We just smiled and said, "No."

After disassembling part of a chair in such a way that maintenance required time and a stocked toolbox to return it to useable status, one nurse was persistent. "What did he do? Before he retired? What did he do?"

He spoke six languages and interrogated prisoners in Vietnam. He carried classified documents, helped a Soviet dissident leave the country, and evaded the KGB on a daily basis. He once negotiated with Chadian drug lords in the desert of North Africa so the United States could get possession of a downed helicopter before the French and Russians got their hands on it. He negotiated a deal to extricate a U.S. military officer out of the Middle East. Then, there was the time he remained on the telephone with a fellow American while a U.S. compound in Africa was overrun.

During that last one, he refused to sleep, even when the line suddenly went dead. He remained alert because the American he had been talking to was a woman, and he knew she would be raped and tortured. He stayed on call until he relocated her, got her medical care in a safe facility, and met with her, face-to-face, to assure she was okay.

He translated and transmitted vital intelligence information and walked some of the most dangerous streets in the world in the Middle East, Central Asia, and Africa. And that was just the stuff we knew about.

"He was in the military." That was all we said.

When he was released from the hospital to a memory-care facility to determine precisely how much brain damage he was suffering from, his wandering truly began. Unlike the hospital, the care facilities did not use restraints, and so our father, though shuffling at a snail's pace, reverted back to his military escape-and-evade tradecraft. He walked in and out of people's rooms as if he belonged there, pulled fire alarms, knocked out a window, and broke the security-code keypad in a tireless effort to discern the number code…twice. His most active times were between two and three in the morning and he would not be re-directed.

Re-direct, we learned, is a super-popular word used in the senior-care world. It means *to distract a senior from what he or she is doing or saying and put them toward another less dangerous or upsetting task.* And in a typical memory-care world, I'm sure re-directing is wildly successful, but when you've spent untold hours, belly down, in the Laos jungles after your plane crashed landed, you've crawled through a darkened cemetery to escape really pissed-off KGB agents who *know* you got the drop on them, or you've remained crouched in a corner, listening to the crackling of far-away voices promising U.S. forces of incoming support, or you've walked among the Hutus and Tootsies following a genocidal bloodbath horrific enough to make international news, re-directing Marc Powe from the task of *not* escaping is pointless. P-o-i-n-t-l-e-s-s.

Usually, he smiled at the person trying to re-direct him then he waited and tried again when they weren't looking. And what worked in his favor? His "captors" distraction with their cell phones. There is a rule in the healthcare world that is both laughable and, apparently, very real. No caregivers are to be on, looking at, using, or even holding their cell phones while on duty.

Let's all take a moment and really, really…*really* laugh.

Feel better?

But seriously, this is a horrible testament to our nation and healthcare system. Caregivers have to be told something that screams *common sense* because they cannot stay away from their phones long enough to make sure fall-risk clients do not do exactly what they are at risk of doing—falling.

Still, their addiction was the perfect scenario for our dad, who, with house slippers ablaze—his ambling pace so swift he could have been lapped by both the hare *and* the tortoise—repeatedly slipped past the preoccupied caregiver toward a new escape route.

The problem with escaping was that he had no real idea where he was going. But he still knew things, somewhere…deep inside. His speech was mostly incoherent—he points and gestures—and full sentences infuriatingly escaped and evaded his own mind. So, he, too, attempted to escape and evade. He pocketed car keys, phones, and purses any chance he got.

"Classic escape and evade tactics," every former military buddy of our father stated.

Still, how do you manage a spy—once considered one of the best in the world—with dementia? It was at this point the caregivers used their phones for more than simply updating their status.

"You need to come take care of your father."

Initially, Michelle took the hardest hit, answering phone calls at 1, 2, and 3 o'clock in the morning.

These five-thousand-a-month facility caregivers declared Daddy "too much to handle" and demanded we bring in additional support when we questioned the frequency of the late-night calls.

What could we do? Daddy couldn't go home. Every physician he'd seen had made that very clear. We had already discovered we couldn't care for our parents ourselves—no matter how hard and long we'd tried. The Veteran's Affairs (VA) had yet to recognize our father's condition, and his long-term healthcare policy wouldn't go into effect until after one hundred and eighty days of active placement within a facility. To repeat—*one hundred and eighty days active placement.*

To make matters worse, our mother's Alzheimer's was accelerating.

At the time, we felt little choice but to come up with another nineteen dollars an hour for an outside service. Daddy needed the care, and we needed the help. Even if it was half-assed, Attila's experience was more than Michelle or I had. Our desperate desire to do whatever was necessary to help our father was our proverbial blood in the water, and sharks like Attila smelled it.

For those keeping track of the math, that calculates to twenty-four-hour rotations with a private sitter service, in addition to the multiple caretakers on staff. Perhaps, that's a better word—care*takers*—because they had no problem helping themselves, over and over and over again, as you'll soon discover. With all the additional help now attending to Daddy's needs, the five thousand going to the facility rapidly racked up to a whopping seventeen thousand dollars a month, and in our situation, the eventual loss of everything. At one point, I worked three different jobs in an attempt to keep up monthly payments, yet these women could not handle one Marc Powe's late-night wandering and mega-speed of turtle-ness.

To add insult to injury, by calling in outside care, the nurses employed by the facility decided it was no longer their job to change our father's diaper—despite the fact that it actually *was* part of their job description and they did so (periodically) for the other residents. The outside aids maintained it was not their job either, and so our father, a man who had dedicated his life to securing peace and would have given his shirt to any of the women had they needed it, was left to sit in diapers so saturated with urine that they sagged to his knees.

Instead of considering how wrong or indignant it was for this man, Attila and company did their own math. They realized we were paying out the nose for all this "care" and concluded we must be rich.

If they only knew!

But their math games made us fair game in their eyes, and that's when they cornered Michelle first, hitting her up for money to cover their own personal expenses.

Yes, you read that correctly.

They aren't dumb, these Attlias.

Had it been me, I would have laughed and set them straight. *I work three jobs. I'm never home. I'm exhausted, and just when I think I might get some sleep, I get a call to come in here at three in the morning to walk at a snail's pace because you won't do your job, but now you want to bleed the turnip even more?!*

I would have let them know my list of demands too. *I want you to do your job. I want to know you are not only taking care of my dad but you are also taking care of the other residents as well. I would like the name and numbers of every family member of the residents here so we can discuss just how much care is really being given.*

The more I thought about it, the more I fantasized. *I am dying to know what your data plan is seeing as you seem to be on that phone nonstop. I would like to turn that thing over to management and let them see how much time you devote to your patients when you're on the clock. Texts alone…Ha!*

I noticed one of the residents down the hall has a saggy diaper, and I wonder…when was she last changed? I wonder how long some of these people sit in urine and fecal matter all day long. I wonder where you were when Ms. Ophelia fell out of her chair.

But Michelle panicked, thinking only of our father. If she said no, would he receive even less

care? While there was no way she could come up with another dollar, she did the best she could

on interrupted sleep, worry, and sheer exhaustion running her brain cells—she stalled.

Thus, our paradox: Daddy's "care" terrified us.

When outsiders learned how we were being bilked, they were enraged on our behalf.

"Refuse to answer the phone at 2 am," they said.

"Report them!"

We tried. The few times we gathered our courage to confront a staff worker or talk to

management, it blew up in our faces. Most care facilities, we discovered, do not want to hear

about residents sitting in saturated diapers yet are slow to correct the situation, as they are afraid

of losing employees.

Case in point—I went to visit our father and found a very sweet, very disoriented female resident

sitting, unattended, in her wheelchair outside the Alzheimer's unit. I stayed, talking with her,

until someone opened the door and then I pushed her inside. Later, when I spoke to the manager,

she had no idea what I was talking about and, while perfectly pleasant, insinuated I was confused

about the dates/times of such an occurrence because "we don't leave people in the hallway."

Ah, but ya did.

But who's going to tell? Certainly not the seniors.

Another sad reality we eventually learned and accepted—until we knew better—is how vastly

over-medicated the residents are. We assumed they were either sleeping or slumped in coma-like

positions because that's what old people did. In actuality, nothing says, "You can talk, play, stare

at your phone for the entire shift," like watching fifteen residents who are stoned out of their

gourds!

Then, there were the times no one slept and phones had to be stuffed away in order to re-direct, verbally and physically. Times when exuberant joy must be quieted and tempers calmed, and Michelle and I recognized early on this was when staff got physical with our dad. Not violent, but physical.

While small in stature, our father is no ninety-eight-pound weakling and there are times he needs physical maneuvering. We understand this. We're okay with this. We've even done it ourselves. *However*, laying hands on him in anger is unacceptable, chiefly because he does not understand what he is doing.

Anger happens. Whether it's in a facility or not, inexplicable feelings of anger and frustration happen quite often when dealing with Alzheimer's and dementia. We get it. We've seen it, time and again, with both our parents as well as many other residents in other facilities. How many times has a resident snapped at me for stealing something I've never seen, moving something that isn't there, being their long-lost daughter, and once, even an old neighbor?

It's not personal. It's dementia.

But when Michelle watched a frustrated caregiver shove our father down, she spoke up.

The aide, accompanied by the facility manager, was confronted by Michelle and, with tremendous attitude, replied, "Well, I'm not sorry because I didn't do anything wrong."

We were paying seventeen thousand a month, losing both sleep and sanity, for *that*?

We moved our father soon after.

Before Daddy's fall, Alzheimer's and dementia weren't even on our radar. Yeah, sure, we knew something was up with Mom, but it's manageable, right? We could kick this thing.

Then, in one day, in one moment, we lost it all. Suddenly, we're looking at startling facts like *the sixth leading cause of death* in this country was Alzheimer's and *there was no cure*. Worse, until recently, so little research had been done because it's considered an "old person's disease" so …

ya know, who really cared?

Things were upside down. This wasn't the highly efficient life Michelle and I grew up in as we

globetrotted and our father saved the world. We grew up knowing our dad was wicked cool, with

access to some of the biggest names in global politics, yet he was unassuming and focused. He

was the perfect blend of powerful, but kind—strong, with a great sense of humanity.

In what felt like the flip of a switch, or the smack of a head on a floor, Daddy was old and

without value or voice. Or so it seemed.

If this could happen to him, what about everyone else? What was happening to those with no

health care at all? What was happening to seniors without daughters to watch over them and help

fight their battles? How had we gone from such a high to this terrible low? Was this how it was

going to be for all of us? The next thing we knew, we're being bullied, ripped off, lied to, and

mishandled.

This was *#LifewithDementia* and our bubble-wrapped world popped with a resounding bang! We

had to reckon with a few things.

There are but two things you can be sure of. First, even if you don't live long enough to become

a senior citizen yourself, you will know and/or love someone who is within your lifetime.

Second, this is our future. All of us.

And so, with those certainties in mind, the family agreed we would tell the whole story—the

good, the bad, the ugly. ***Operation Caregivers: #LifewithDementia*** is the story we would have

much preferred to have read than lived, but we are so very grateful for the information we have

and believe it is our duty to share. Our dad would have wanted it this way.

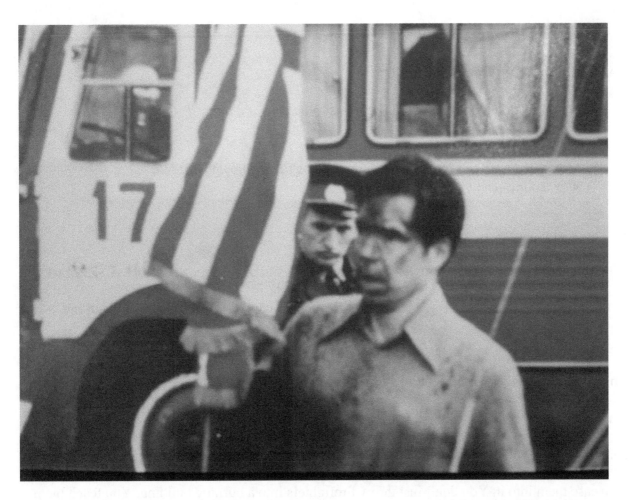

Lieutenant Colonel Powe saved the American flag from burning...much to the disapproval of the Soviet guard behind him

Chapter Two

FACEBOOK POST: *Thanksgiving 2016*

> *Alex: Well, this is nice, and Daddy seems to be enjoying himself.*
> *Mom: Where is your father?*
> *Michelle: Mom, he's sitting right next to you.*
> *Mom: Oh. Well, this is nice, and Daddy seems to be enjoying himself.*
> *Alex: Funny echo in here...*

Everyone approaches aging differently.

When I opened the mailbox on my birthday and discovered a welcome card from AARP, I was most intrigued to learn I had earned a free AARP pouch, which I use to this day to haul my music around for the various cardio classes I teach.

Michelle, on the other hand, went into a mild rage and swore vengeance against the PR person who desecrated her day of birth and gift-getting with an age-reminding slap in the face. "It's completely insensitive and stupid. You have to let someone come to grips with first being fifty. You ease them into it. You don't just throw firefighters into a burning building. You teach them how to approach the fire! This is the same thing. I needed more time!"

Michelle does not own a really cool AARP black pouch. But she does possess a giant chip on her fifty-(plus) year-old shoulder.

Then again, for as much as we have in common, we've always approached life differently. Professionally, Michelle teaches English. She holds a master's in English literature and loves the classics, with their dark, brooding characters filled with despair, remorse, and regret. The only reason I don't stab out my eardrums so I won't have to listen is because they truly bring her happiness. She is always the most popular teacher at whatever campus she sets up on and always gives more time to her students than she actually has. She is also funny, and her students adore her and so, apparently, they have also chosen not to stab out their eardrums so that they may hear all about the stories that so enchant Ms. Powe.

While Michelle deals primarily with teenagers and young adults, my students range in age from early twenties to mid-nineties. I teach kinesiology at a local community college and depending upon the student, some might say my classes are more torturous than Emily Bronte or Virginia Wolfe or Toni Morrison combined. Beyond torturing millennials—a fun gig, if you can get it—I also teach Silver Sneakers and the special needs.

It is with the senior population that I have learned the most. This group is so varied because of both age and range of functional movement. My students are there for medical reasons ranging from diabetes, heart condition, scoliosis, and double knee replacement to stroke, Parkinson's (early stages), rheumatoid arthritis, and obesity. But many more are there simply because they understand that maintaining health means staying active, retaining as much bone density and muscle as possible, as well as proper blood circulation, and socialization. That last one is a biggie. It is my job, and one I take seriously—to motivate and inspire. Along with so many other issues, depression and anxiety is a growing concern with many of my students.

Michelle also battles depression. Hers has been a series of bad decisions leading to bad results and, for a time, it almost swallowed her whole. All of these aspects are important to note since I approach my own parents' plummeting health and abilities differently than my sister.

Too many Americans view age as a flaw. As long as you are young and beautiful and can perform one hundred jump squats, you have value. I can't count the number of times, in my own gym, I heard other people make snarky comments about *the blue hairs*, aka the elderly.

But I know better.

As a group, they are energetic, socially active, and fun. After class, and even during sometimes, the Silver Sneakers and I have conversations ranging from health, nutrition, and functional movement to local news, social responsibilities, family, and communal efforts. This is the group that best represents what fitness is. They are hungry for knowledge about heart health, bone density, muscle development, balance, functional movement, proper form, and better nutrition. But they are also extremely invested in the idea of cognitive training, keeping their wits sharp, and working memory skills. They understand how important it is to exercise the brain as much as the body.

I am routinely inspired by their personal stories. Collectively, they are cancer survivors, widows(ers), and are constantly challenged by various other medical issues that, instead of shutting them down, have made them more determined than ever to stay as strong as possible for as long as possible. As I watch their movements, I find little nuggets of information from each one that have me redefining strength, courage, and determination, but also health, wellness, and what happiness really means. I see those who are living life well. It is a shame so many instructors do not want to train the older population due to misguided beliefs that they are limited in movement and strength. In reality, this subset of our society makes instructors better for everyone, of *all* ages.

Before all hell broke loose in my parents' lives, I was begging and pleading for them to come to the gym. I *knew* the benefits of being physically fit. I saw the benefits. I saw how energized the Silver Sneaker class was, how they built true friendships in the class, and how they checked on one another if someone skipped a few classes. I wanted that for my parents. As much as Mom was struggling with day-to-day activities, I knew in my heart this could help her!

So, when we got them moved, I arranged free gym memberships for my parents and even suggested they take class with another teacher. My mother's pride was mighty, and I realized that she might feel better with someone other than her daughter instructing her. But it was one excuse after another why they could not come.

Mom took moving the hardest. She claimed she hated Texas and blamed our father for dragging her here—her children, grandchildren, free gym memberships, and Silver Sneakers socializing be damned. She was confused, disoriented, and scared. For her, this manifested in unforgiving, whirling anger.

We couldn't understand the anger at the time but, in hindsight, now know that a geographical change for anyone with Alzheimer's and/or dementia is crushing. Mom was as good a con artist as our father and, in many ways, I suppose, that's why they were so perfect for each other from the start. While our father came from very humble means, Mom was a princess. Her father was a very successful country club manager who, always in demand, travelled around the south to whip country clubs back into shape. Mom grew up with maids, chauffeurs, cooks, and various others taking care of things. It was during the 1940s and 50s, and most of Mom's exposure to blacks was as "the help." Specifically, *her* help. She had (and sometimes still has) extremely fond memories of them all. And so, the 60s were a bit of a shock when, as a young adult, she realized there were white people who didn't like black people; there were black people who thought working at a country club, doting on a little white girl, might be demeaning; perhaps the staff she had always known and loved were there not out of love for working in country clubs but out of necessity.

Many years ago, I asked her outright. "Mom, did it not occur to you that it would suck to work for a country club that would never allow you to be a member because of the color of your skin?"

It had not. At least, as a child, she had not seen it that way.

After our parents married and our father began his career in military intelligence, Mom found her cause. We had been assigned to Baltimore, Maryland, and Mom learned a re-zoning of voting districts had made it difficult for the black populace to make it to the voting polls.

She gathered all one hundred and twelve pounds of her indignant, yet mighty, self, loaded my sister and me in the car, and began driving out to the poorest sections of Baltimore to transport voters to the polls.

It was in this same bad section of town, a young black man approached Mom as she was getting into her car and demanded her purse.

Mom whirled—

Now, see, I know I'm a writer and may be given to more dramatic descriptions for better storytelling but, honestly, Karen Powe whirls. She's been a whirler since the day she was donning frilly white dresses and stamping her patent-leather shoes on the greens of her father's country club lawns. So…

She whirled on this young man. "Does your mother know where you are?"

Stunned, he walked away without another word.

But we—Michelle and I—know what really happened. We've seen it our entire lives. Karen Powe is this little tiny woman, with large brown eyes and pip-squeak arms that couldn't wrestle open a can of worms, even with an electric screwdriver, but when she's mad, she radiates danger.

A rattlesnake is quite small but can be terrifying. That's Mom. There's something about her. When she whirls on you, the response is primal—Retreat! Retreat! The tiny woman is whirling! In 2014, after their move, Mom whirled on our dad. She hated Texas. She wanted to go back home, to Virginia. It didn't matter that they had no family—only a handful of friends from the military days—there. It didn't matter that her grandchildren were here, and she could see us more often than she had in an entire decade. She was leaving!

The irony was that, even though she was dead-set on leaving the state of Texas, she refused to leave the house.

Of course, *now* we recognize that for what it is.

More than a decade ago, Mom stopped going to any functions with our father, she stopped doing the grocery shopping, and if she did go out, it was a major event.

Then, five years ago, our parents got a dog, and while we initially believed the dog would make great company for Mom, Colby turned out to be a crutch. The sweet oversized Labra-Dane (a mix between a Labrador retriever and Great Dane) our parents got while still living in D.C. had been neglected and was in need of serious TLC. Mom fretted and fussed over him, and by the time they moved to Texas, every conversation, phone call, and story she took part in was about Colby.

My sister and I have always been *big time* dog lovers, but this was annoying. Even so, we accepted that Mom didn't think she could go shopping, see a movie, eat out, or go to the gym because she couldn't leave Colby. Colby was her addiction, her obsession, and we did not yet know enough about Alzheimer's or dementia to understand he was the cover for her dementia. He was also her security blanket, and the one sense of control she had left.

Our dad, on the other hand, had always been super social and so staying holed up in the house with Colby was simply not an option for him. So, he ran errands. He made as many as two or three trips into town a day. He found reasons to go to the post office, Home Depot, and the bookstore. Unlike Mom, Daddy very much wanted to go to the gym, and he searched for ways to make it happen.

"Do they have a daycare there?" he asked during one of our calls.

I looked at the phone. *Oh, no.* "Yesss," I said slowly. *Surely, he's not going to sugges—*

"Would they take a dog?"

How to play this? My mind raced. *Do I say yes just to get them in the door and secretly hire a college student to walk Colby around the outside perimeter of the gym the entire time they are working out? How do I smuggle a hundred-pound Labra-Dane into the gym? Does Colby know how to do bicep curls? Does Colby have biceps?*

I wish now, knowing all that we've learned, I'd said, "Daddy, we have to stop doing backflips for Mom. It's not helping." I wish I had pointed out the obvious—Mom's mental health is rapidly deteriorating.

But I didn't. Instead, I simply said, "I don't think so, Daddy."

We knew things were happening that weren't good, but asking too many questions angered our mother, and Michelle and I were caught up in the game of pretend. While Michelle was in straight-up denial, I was busily comparing my parents to my Silver Sneakers students and how I thought my parents *should be* in ability and stability.

They no sooner got moved to Texas than Mom began showing signs we weren't able to see over the phone. She put toothpaste in the food pantry, crackers in the living room, and razors with the cups and glasses. Mom couldn't seem to remember to close the refrigerator door, and it seemed impossible to grasp that all the Tupperware was hers. But it was more than that. She was

suddenly a collector—from plastic bags to McDonalds' straws to bottle tops and more.

As Michelle logically attempted to place all the pans together, Mom whirled, and I lingered in

the background, whispering, "She's whirling! Watch out. She's whirling!"

Michelle, with obsessive tendencies all her own, could not let things go and pushed for towels to

be placed in the linen closet or Tupperware in the kitchen until Mom would sic Daddy on us.

We tried talking to our father, but he was obsessed with calls and incoming mail from

Washington, so we refocused on our mom again, trying desperately to get permission to help her

with unpacking. We were typically given a grace period of about thirty minutes before our

activity became overwhelming for Mom and she ordered us out of the house.

If we could just get Mom outside those four walls, we were sure she would be so much happier.

Again and again, I tried to tell her about the men and women in the Silver Sneakers program, but

she would not hear it. Instead, she focused on Colby…or the past, which took on the face of an

old friend from Ohio.

Patricia Caston, a former Buckeye neighbor of mine, became part of our family in the mid-90s,

after she and Michelle traveled to Poland together to teach English while my younger daughters

and I took care of her cats. Ms. Pat, already in her late seventies when she went overseas, was a

phenomenal hit with the international kids as she had only one volume and one channel—loud

and shocking.

Once they returned to the States, Ms. Pat met our mother and they became fast friends.

So it made sense, when Ms. Pat moved into a retirement community, Mom would visit. A bit of a

social butterfly back in the day, and then in her mid-sixties, Mom became buddies with women

in their late eighties and early nineties. For reasons we could not understand, Mom adapted and, it seemed almost overnight, was suddenly quite elderly. And she wanted nothing more than to move there, surrounded by Pat and her other new friends.

The only stand our father ever took against our mom was his refusal to move to Ohio to live in that retirement community.

As much as it hurt us, my children included, at the time—our mother, their grandmother, would rather live in a retirement home in Ohio among (mostly) strangers than next door to us in Texas—we see now how much Mom wanted to hide from the world. If she was with other elderly people, no explanations were needed as to why she had no idea how to operate a stove or work at teakettle or turn on a garden hose.

I finally managed to get my parents into the gym, and while my father looked impressed, intrigued, even excited, Mom had a look of smoldering rage. She was going to whirl at any moment.

We walked toward Fitness Room #1 where a Silver Sneakers class was ongoing. I wanted to show my mother how big the class was, how cool and fun everyone was.

As soon as some of the members in the class saw me standing outside, they waved, and several left their chairs to come say hi.

"Are these your parents?" they asked.

As proud as I was to show my parents and the Silver Sneakers off, I was embarrassed and a little confused why Mom was being such a little snot. She was more than aloof. She barely made eye contact with anyone and made it painfully clear that she would not be staying, much less attend a fitness class.

That was the first and last time Mom set foot in my gym. When did Mom become such a brat? So unsocial? So old?

Michelle and I found ourselves asking those questions and more a lot. *When did the pack-rat behavior begin? When did she start putting everything in Ziploc baggies? And since when was she sponsoring a Native American tribe in Utah?*

A web article regarding senior citizens and signs of dementia caught my attention. Beyond the symptoms, many of which we had already looked at, there were also cautionary words about how the elderly hide those signs. "No longer willing to participate in social gatherings or activities they once did…"

Well, we were already there.

It made sense why our father stopped letting us talk to Mom on the phone, but now that we were face-to-face every day, we also saw that Daddy was preparing all the meals, doing all the grocery shopping, and Mom no longer drove. In fact, Mom no longer got online and hadn't for more than five years, even though our dad still insisted people "include Mom on emails, please."

What? Why?

One day, we were standing outside the house, and I broke down and asked. "Daddy, why ask people to include Mom on emails when she doesn't get on the computer, hasn't for years and, honestly, has no clue how to even turn it on?"

"I'll take that under advisement," he said.

"You'll take that under advi—" *What the heck is he talking about?*

It was the beginning of 2015, and every day was Groundhog Day with Mom. She was on a train track of dialogue that went 'round and 'round in a circle. But it wasn't just the same stories over and over. She was repeating herself, almost verbatim, within mere minutes—even seconds—with zero memory of having just shared the story. She lined every pocket with dog kibble, placed bags within bags, and would fly into near rages if and when Michelle or I tried to bring order to the growing chaos of their home. And something smelled. Something always smelled—wrong.

In a mind-blowing story that, for my own sanity, I will make very short, Michelle took one for the team and flew with Mom back to Ohio. Mom wanted to see Ms. Pat so a plane ticket was booked by our father.

What was intended to be a one-time plane trip to Ohio ended up spanning two weeks and three separate attempts, with a total of six trips to and from the airport, including two taxi rides—at one hundred bucks a pop—back to the house with Mom, and both times leaving our father standing in the airport. Unbeknownst at the time, Mom's dementia was so great that the moment she stepped inside the hustle and bustle of the airport, she would walk away from our father, who was checking her luggage for her. When Daddy turned his back, Mom panicked, walked out of the airport, hailed a taxi, and read off the address she had written on a piece of paper she had placed in her pocket.

And here's the kicker: We later learned Daddy had also made several erroneous ticket purchases and tried to give a security guard Mom's luggage. It wasn't just Mom. It was Daddy, too!

We pleaded with our father to stop trying to send Mom to Ohio. Especially since he had purchased tickets with a layover in Chicago.

My God, we would lose her forever! How could he not see sending Mom off alone to another airport could not *happen?*

"I think he's trying to kill Mom," Michelle said.

We chuckled about it at the time, but only a little because—hindsight is great—I swear, it seemed as if he really *was* trying to kill Mom. What we initially believed to be denial on our father's part was the beginnings of his own dementia.

At last, Michelle, unable to stand the idea of Mom traveling alone, purchased her own ticket as well.

A mere eight hours after landing in Ohio, at two in the morning, Mom repacked her bags and was standing at Ms. Pat's front door, believing she had just spent a week there, and it was time to leave.

By the second night, Michelle called me from a stairwell in the retirement community. "I. Hate. You."

"What? Why?"

"Because. You let me come here."

Mom and a then ninety-two-year-old Ms. Pat were getting loaded on boxed wine while Mom accused Michelle and me of stealing her money.

Michelle knew it was garbage, but it still hurt. She had taken off time from work to safely transport Mom to see her buddy, and all Mom had done was make accusations and vicious remarks about Michelle from the minute they got there.

"She doesn't know what she's saying." I repeated that phrase to Michelle again and again, but it still hurt.

We had to learn how to ignore the comments.

After five days, Mom's anxiety had grown to epic proportions. She had worn the same clothes every day, insisting that was the day she was leaving. Needless to say, it was a wild and exhausting trip.

By spring, red flags were popping all over the place. Mom still made passing comments about moving back to Virginia, but now both parents were being weirdly secretive and, for the first time in years, our concerns shifted from Mom to our father. He couldn't hold a thought, forgot words, and kept getting lost.

The man was legendary for navigating his way around hostile countries but couldn't find the grocery store?! He had navigated his way out of a jungle, out of a foreign country without GPS, and had retraced his tracks to a safe house in an unknown city, yet now he got lost going from Point A to Point B with a map!

He was never the type of father who sat and played games with his children. Heck, he was rarely home, but we, even as children, understood he was off doing important things, like saving the world and stuff.

The one time he actively participated in our lives was during high school, when he coached our soccer team, but he became too intense. He took coaching to the extreme. So much so that most of the team threatened to quit before the season ever really started unless Mom took over. Seriously, how many sixteen-year-old girls really want to be in a military boot camp complete with soccer balls flying at their heads?

That example aside, Daddy had always been polite, always patient, and always willing to talk about a problem or have a laugh.

Now, however, he constantly interrupted. It wasn't just with us, but with people in stores, other family members, neighbors, or some stranger in line. It didn't seem to matter. He interrupted and/or spoke over everyone, not having heard a single word anyone else said.

I couldn't decide it if was that he didn't hear or that he simply didn't care.

We urged him to get his hearing aids checked at the VA in Dallas.

When he became obsessed with his laptop, constantly checking emails and muttering about people in Washington, Michelle and I were confused.

When our father retired from the military, he moved into the private sector and quickly got a job in New York City as head security chief for the United Nations. The position sent him around the world, and by the time his service with the UN was up, he had visited every single nation within the African continent at least twice. Next came the Pentagon's Assistant Director of African Affairs as his grasp of French and Arabic were still strong, but even more, Daddy loved the people of the Middle East and Africa. He was 'da man to talk to when it came to Middle Eastern, African, and Russian affairs.

By 2010, he was having difficulties at his newest post. It was with another national security firm—the name and location were never disclosed—and his boss didn't like him. We were shocked. Who didn't like Marc Powe? Everyone—excluding a few teenaged girls for a brief time during soccer season—loved him. But Mom told us stories about how this new young staff didn't think the Colonel knew what he was talking about or what he was doing. Essentially, he was forced out of the job in the most kind and polite way possible, and we chalked it up to new kids on the block taking over the helm.

But now, seeing and hearing him on a daily basis, things were becoming clearer.

One particularly telling moment came during a call from him.

"Hi, honey. Do you have room for me to put some meat in your deep freezer?"

"Sure. How much meat?" I was curious. After all, my parents were small people who barely ate. I mean…Mom's downright *tiny*. How much meat could they possibly have?

"Oh, about two large boxes worth."

"Mm-hm. Where's Mom?" Just checking. Listen, after hearing the same gosh-dern story about Colby and a squirrel, I was ready to kill Mom and I didn't live with her. But, no, Mom was safe and sound.

Sure enough, when I went to retrieve the meat there were two boxes of every kind, from BBQ pork to regular pork chops, supposedly steak (which is awful, by the way), variations of seasoned and plain chicken (which we actually suspect to be something else), and ground beef.

Apparently, "two nice young men" selling meat from their truck had knocked on his door, and Daddy had bought it. Hook, line, and seven hundred and fifty dollars' worth of meat sinker.

Sufficiently appalled, I was also speechless. I wanted to chastise him for being so gullible, but he was my dad. I couldn't. I was mortified on his behalf. Could he not see how wrong this was? I was all over the Better Business Bureau because, and I still ask, how could "two nice young men" honestly believe two of the tiniest adults you'd ever meet could eat that much animal protein?

Just the week before, he'd paid a local shop over nine hundred and fifty dollars to get Mom's laptop "repaired."

When I saw the receipt I asked Mom, "Are you getting on the computer these days?"

She looked at me like I was speaking Swahili, and my concerns about money being spent hand over fist grew.

But back to the meat wagon.

When I found my voice, I tried to broach the idea that maybe he had spent too much money on this much meat. There was no way he or Mom could possibly eat it all and maybe—

But he was already talking about Washington D.C. again. They needed him. They were constant. They wouldn't leave him alone.

That stopped me. "What do you mean they won't leave you alone?"

As I've mentioned, we'd heard these utterances before but thought nothing of them. Daddy had frequently spoken to high-ranking officials, foreign dignitaries, politicians, and such during his years with the military and well after. But standing in his driveway, looking at hundreds of dollars' worth of unidentifiable meat in my trunk, clarity seemed really important.

"*Who* won't leave you alone?"

He sighed. "Barack Obama and Hillary."

Um. Okay.

Our dad had chatted with Kennedys and the Reagans, he'd worked with Colin Powell and other big wigs, but that had been then.

Now, he was standing in Waxahachie, Texas, and the biggest thing he had going were his daily trips to CVS because he thought it was funny to heckle the pharmacist who was a Longhorn. Daddy was an Aggie. The idea of Hillary and Barack sending him personal emails was … unlikely.

Yet, willing to give the benefit of the doubt, I persisted. "What do they want?"

"My help!"

I sought out my mother. "Mom, Daddy thinks Barack Obama is sending him personal emails."

With big eyes and a bright smile, Mom nodded. "He is."

I tried to reason with her, but this was a slippery slope because we'd all met Barack Obama before. We had shaken his hand, taken pictures with him, and he'd even chatted with my son.

I tried another tactic by pointing out that, as busy as the president was, it was highly improbable he had time to email anyone outside the Beltway, particularly one retired and now living in Texas.

Mom's response was retrieving two framed letters for my inspection.

"These are the communications?"

Mom looked so pleased, and it really was a horrible moment. Not because Mrs. Clinton and Mr. Obama weren't really contacting my father, but because my parents both believed them to be legitimate personal letters. In fact, they were standard flush letters sent to the masses, but with a "personal" greeting made possible only in recent years with new technology.

Both letters read: "Marc—I need your help!" The plea was followed by statements pertaining to how Daddy's financial contributions to a political campaign could save the world.

It was the first time in my life I wrestled with a horrible fact that my father had no idea what was going on. It was also the first time I became familiar with the word *anosognosia*. Until that moment, my sister and I thought my father was in total denial about our mother's condition but it was more. Much more.

Anosognosia means *to be completely unaware of impairment*. With anatomical changes or damage to the brain, researchers have determined a patient can be unaware of his or her own illness, and Daddy was suffering. Mom knew something was wrong with her, and so she went out of her way to hide it or simply bit our heads off to deflect our interest in her inabilities, but Daddy…Daddy had no clue.

The horrible truth was that he was far more destructive than Mom. Daddy was very capable with the computer and his credit cards, and because he thought he was on another mission, he was a dangerous, dangerous man.

Oh, and lest I forget, he had also become obsessed with the idea of winning five thousand dollars a month for the rest of his life through Publishers Clearing House.

Ho, boy. *Operation Shut-Daddy-Down* was set in motion.

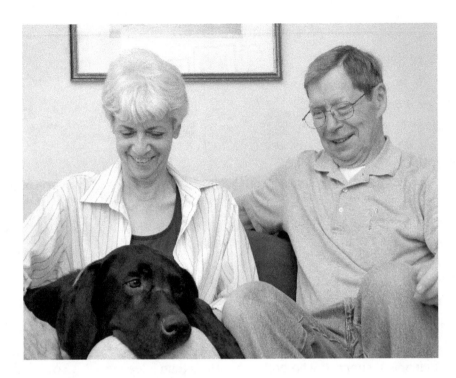

Living outside Washington D.C., Marc and Karen adopted Colby, the Labor-Dane, who stole their hearts (and annoyed everyone else's)

Chapter Three

July 2017

> *Alex: Knock. Knock.*
> *Mom: [blank stare]*
> *Alex: No. Mom, it's a joke. Okay, ready? Knock. Knock.*
> *Mom: What?*
> *Alex: No, who. I say, 'Knock, knock,' and you say, 'Who's there.' Okay, ready? Knock.*
>   *Knock.*
> Mom: [a little uncertainly] Who's there?
> Alex: Cow says.
> Mom: What?
> Alex: No, I say, 'Cow says' and you say, 'Cow says who.'
> Mom: Cow says mooo
> Alex: You're killin' me, Mom. You're killin' me.

When in need of technical support, who better to turn to than a teenager? As our dad madly downloaded letters sent to him by senators, congressmen and women, Hillary, Barack Obama, more than a dozen organizations for various political platforms, a number of United Nations, Red Cross, and other groups that served women and children in the Middle Eastern and African regions, I got Tommy, my then-fifteen-year old son, to hack into my dad's email account.

Any guilt I felt about sneaking into my father's account was assuaged the moment his email page opened before me. Literally hundreds of emails were addressed to my father with similar greetings.

"I need your help, Marc."

"Thank you, Marc, for making a difference."

"Dear Marc, we need you…"

It was stunning.

It was sickening.

Vultures descended upon my father, in record numbers, as one-time contributions were not

enough. Congressmen and women, U.S. Senators, and political hopefuls from across the nation

littered his email box. How did a man, previously from Virginia, now living in Texas, have so

much correspondence from Indiana, Illinois, Florida, North Dakota, California, Ohio, and

Washington state?

Hundreds and hundreds of dollars had been given to a Tammy Duckworth in Illinois alone, and

the dollar sums given to Hillary Clinton's campaign were almost as mind-numbing as the

number of requests begging my father for more help, more support, more money.

Again and again I saw something called Act Blue in his emails. Act Blue not only acted as the

debt collector to these contributions but it also charged a small fee for the trouble. Over and over

they thanked my dad for the contribution of twenty, twenty-five, thirty-five, fifty-five dollars.

I called Act Blue.

I had no legal rights, no Power of Attorney, just desperation.

Initially, the man scoffed when I said that it appeared my father was making donations to every

senator and representative in every state. After a quick review, however, he whistled in disbelief.

It turned out that he had indeed made contributions to every senator and representative of every

state who had made a request of him.

In one of the few positive experiences in which an organization/company was taking money

from our parents, Act Blue moved swiftly once it realized what was happening.

After begging a manager to simply review our father's account, a perfectly lovely human being

came back to say, "I don't think your father understand how this works." It was explained that,

normally, a person started one account with one credit card and made various contributions from

that single account/credit card.

Our dad, never one to do anything half-assed, had set up numerous accounts using various credit cards, with automatically recurring contributions, no less.

We learned that, in just ten months, Daddy had given over thirty thousand dollars in contributions. That figure didn't include what he had also given to PBS, The Children's Fund, UNICEF, United Nations, three Native American Indian tribes in Utah, North Dakota, and Arizona, and a variety of other organizations.

The number, at last count, could be as high as fifty thousand during that same ten-month period.

Picture it: *Operation Deletion Day* (aka Op D-Day: Act Blue). I needed my father preoccupied and *not* looking at his computer while I erased every one of his automatically withdrawing Act Blue accounts and their corresponding emails. My eldest, Kerri, had come home for a visit so I sent her to her grandparents as the perfect distraction.

In true military-brat tradition, the objectives were stated. "Your mission, should you choose to accept it, is to make sure Papa does not look at his laptop for at least thirty minutes. Do you accept?"

Kerri nodded and headed off for *Operation Distract Papa* so that I could exact *Operation Deletion.*

Two hours later, she came home sweaty.

I never really asked why she was sweating, but the mission was a success!

Unfortunately, *Operation Deletion* didn't last long and, soon enough, he was back at it.

In hindsight, I wish I had been more forthcoming. Maybe Daddy would have listened.

Probably not.

I reached out to some old friends of my parents, asking them to throw out hints about giving money away, but he heard nothing.

Quite literally. Not only was he tuning out the world over his obsession with the Internet and giving, he was not putting in his hearing aids. And he rarely spoke, especially to Mom, but that seemed to be an even trade because she barely spoke, period. When she did, it was in a whispered voice so soft that Michelle and I, after insisting she force something louder than a mouse fart from her throat, began wondering if we needed hearing aids as well.

While Mom whispered her way through life, denying her husband was spending too much time on the Internet and giving away too much money, I woke every morning at 5 am, logged onto my father's account and stopped every contribution he'd made in the past twenty-four hours before jumping over to the trash account and deleting any evidence I'd been there. As fast as he spent, I was unsubscribing him from the politicians' newsletters.

They were a savvy bunch, however, and as quickly as I clicked *unsubscribe*, they sent out more urgent notes.

"Marc! We need you!"

"Marc, you are making a difference."

"Marc, we can't do this without you!"

The last became my personal favorite as I began sending scathing notes back to them as if I were Marc Powe.

Yeah, well, you're gonna have to because my daughter is getting really pissed and is about to send an open letter to the Wall Street Journal *and* New York Times *about how you prey on the elderly, knowing they are on a fixed income, but make them believe they have to give up their house to pay for your campaign!*

Funny, Daddy never got a single reply back from those emails.

As the months wore on, I grew bolder in my exchanges. I kept warning myself I was going to get caught. It was only a matter of time. But I was ready. If he confronted me, I would merely show him all the back and forth email exchanges exposing the hundreds and hundreds—nay, *thousands* of dollars he was giving away.

But he never caught on.

It is essential I make something perfectly clear. As of this writing, I know of just as many stories of the Republican party preying on the elderly. It is both dangerous and destructive to believe that one party is more aggressive than another in its quest for campaign contributions. Politicians are a different beast. They will take money any way they can get it, regardless of which side of the aisle they or your loved one is on, and care very little that your loved one is on a fixed income. In fact, in recent years, scare tactics have become the popular go-to in persuading the elderly to contribute more.

Businesses are no better.

Through a friend, I learned of a woman who was literally spending thousands on QVC. Her family sent doctors' reports and Power of Attorney notifications, asking QVC to refuse her credit card purchases, but the company maintained it was her right as an American citizen to purchase whatever she wanted—despite medical reports showing she had Alzheimer's.

While Daddy didn't much care for QVC, he was all over the Internet.

I discovered that Publishers Clearing House (PCH) was one of the most aggressive, and Daddy, convinced that "$5,000 a week for life" win was just a few clicks away, responded in kind. I repeatedly unsubscribed but PCH wanted its money…just a little bit more.

When I found subscriptions confirmations for a number of magazines, I went in search of the titles. "Mom! Why are you getting Golf Digest? Daddy has never golfed a single day in his life!"

"I know. It's the strangest thing. These magazines just keep coming," she said, sounding as dismayed as I.

I tried to explain that they were coming because Daddy was subscribing to them but she just laughed.

"Oh, honey, don't be ridiculous. Why would your father subscribe to a golf magazine? He's never play golf in his life."

Sigh. *Well, ya got me there.*

In addition to his new monthly fascination with all things golf was the inexplicable arrival of *US Weekly* every Tuesday. Colonel Marc Powe—a man who would rather set himself on fire than talk about celebrities and "what's hot" in Hollywood—had a sudden desire for a gossip rag? He was always a sharp-dressed man, so maybe that explained why he needed *GQ*. And while he had never fished a day in his life, viewing it as something for idle hands, apparently, he was also dying to read the latest copy of *Field and Stream*.

I called the PCH call center.

For more than ten minutes, I went around and around with a representative. I acknowledged that Daddy subscribed but explained he didn't understand what he was doing, and I asked that they remove his name from their contact list.

The rep said PCH wasn't responsible for what people signed up for and that maybe my father really *wanted* these magazines.

I was beyond frustrated. "He is a 5'7", thin, white, *elderly* man! Do you really think he wants a hip-hop basketball magazine?" The only hip the man had to his hop was a fractured one if he tried to jump.

Publishers Clearing House was unmoved, and it would take another three months before I finally

shut them down even a little. We still got *Men's Fitness, Entrepreneur, Inc.*, and *Wired* along

with several other magazines for another ten months.

I kept a strict policy when trolling Daddy's emails, at first. If it appeared personal, I wouldn't

open it, but as time went on, with more politicians presenting themselves as a pal, a buddy, one

of the guys, I began reading more and more. (Sincerest apologies to anyone reading this now

who once sent a social note to my father. My intentions weren't to pry but to keep his best

interests at heart.) That was when I came across one of several conversations between Daddy,

two real estate agents, a financial broker, and a friend discussing the fact that he and Karen

(Mom) would be moving back to the D.C. area in the spring of 2016.

I felt I danced near another line when I contacted many of those mentioned and asked them not

to encourage the move, as it was dangerous.

I gave in and jumped that invisible line when I revealed a few of the medical concerns Michelle

and I were having, but something had to be said.

I also began telling family and friends what I was doing in an effort to maintain full disclosure. I

explained going into Daddy's email every day, throughout the day, and checking excessive

spending. I thought it important that other family members and friends knew what was really

happening. Daddy never knew what I was doing.

I guess that was the point, though, wasn't it? He wasn't catching anything.

He was, however, walking Colby nonstop.

With Mom tipping the scales at ninety-eight pounds and Daddy at approximately one hundred

and thirty, a strong northerly wind could knock them both off course. Colby, though sweet in nature, never understood his size and had a tendency to pull on the leash. I was convinced Colby was going to kill one of them!

Both Michelle and I begged them to stop walking Colby as they had a perfectly nice fenced-in yard, but Mom declared Colby did not like the yard. No, walking within range of every barking dog and squirrel in the neighborhood seemed a much better idea to her.

Oh, and ducks. Did I mention the ducks?

One of the many purposes of this book is to use our hindsight as a spotlight for someone else. So many of our sentences these days begin with, "Oh, *that's* why that was happening…"

The topic of dog walking is no different.

We could not understand why Mom was being so difficult. It didn't matter if it was melt-your-face-off hot or if it was raining. Colby couldn't use his backyard. It didn't help matters that Daddy appeared to be getting clumsier, even commenting himself that his balance seemed off. But Mom dug in, saying that she would walk Colby instead.

Oh, yeah. Sure. That's much more reasonable.

But the more we tried to reason with her about safety issues, the more firmly she planted her heels.

Daily, they walked Colby to the duck pond and back…because nothing could go wrong with that plan.

In addition to the potential ski trip Colby might take my parents on, there was also my parents' neighbor—diagnosed with Alzheimer's and everything—whose wife allowed him to drive the neighborhood "because it makes him happy."

What?

When I repeated this bit of horror to my Silver Sneakers class, many nodded. That wasn't unusual. They informed me this was typical with older couples who wanted to see the other happy—despite a diagnosis of dementia and/or Alzheimer's, which allowed for at least the possibility of the other driving off into the sunset never to return or, worse, mowing over a group of kids—or a couple walking their Labra-Dane—on the sidewalk!

The common denominator: *I love my spouse so I will allow for this behavior because it makes him/her happy and I'll just cross my fingers that nothing bad happens.*

For Mom and Daddy, it was a show of independence, which made them happy.

Mom truly hates being told she *can't* or *shouldn't* do something, especially if it's something she once did. She has always been a stubborn woman, but as she has lost more and more control over her own memory and thoughts, she clings to whatever she can as a show of empowerment. Of course, she didn't walk Colby but a few times, but the fact that she *could* was all she needed.

It was early fall of 2015, but still very hot in Texas, when I came in the house to find Daddy sitting at the kitchen table, staring into the distance, with Colby sprawled out on the marble floor, panting happily, and I made one of those lame jokes. "Who walked whom?"

Daddy just stared at me.

I almost laughed before I realized he was in distress. Having worked in the fitness industry for over twenty-five years, with specializations in senior citizens and the special needs, I knew that look. He was powering down—and not in a good way. "Daddy! Daddy? Can you hear me? Can you talk?"

He had nothing left to give but a blank stare.

I quickly placed fingertips on his carotid artery, thinking I would do a count but it wasn't needed. His pulse was through the roof. "Mom? How long has he been like this?"

She was completely and utterly clueless.

I pointed at Daddy. "Look at him!"

Hers became a mirrored expression of blankness.

My, God!

I later told my sister they couldn't take care of each other. It was the first true reckoning we'd had on that topic. We'd deluded ourselves into thinking, as insane as all of Daddy's spending and Mom's hoarding was, that they still, somehow, had each other's backs. Obviously, that was no longer true.

She must have walked passed Daddy a dozen times after he got home, even spoken to him, but they both dwelled in their own worlds.

I got him in the car and took him to the ER. That was when I learned not only how bad Daddy's heart really was but also that Mom had no clue about his medical history. She knew nothing.

Mom didn't know Daddy's birth date.

Mom didn't know her address.

Mom didn't know what day it was.

I looked at her. Either I was the dumbest daughter on the planet or she had masterfully learned to adapt, to act as though she knew more of what was going on the less she knew.

I called Michelle, our family medical expert, to fill in the blanks. When Michelle arrived and we reviewed our father's history with a pacemaker and how erratic his heartbeat was, it was agreed—he needed to stay overnight for observation. He was sedated for a series of tests and set up with a private room.

With the Ohio trip still fresh in our minds, we *really* hesitated when Mom announced she would also spend the night with her husband.

Once again, Michelle took one for the team and agreed to stay in the hospital room with our parents.

Mom fussed over Daddy well into the night, but about midnight—a full hour after Mom had fallen asleep—Michelle thought it was safe to go home, take care of her dogs and, perhaps, get a few hours of sleep before heading back to work. I was coming in at six, after all. Where's the harm?

But at 2 o'clock that morning, the Waxahachie Baylor Hospital called Michelle to come get her mother.

As it turned out, it took less than two hours for Mom to wake, pack their belongings, and rouse our still-drugged father from his sleep because she had decided they had to go home. With the keys in her hands, but no knowledge how to drive or where exactly their home was, she thought it best that Daddy drive them.

When the nurses saw our father stumbling and staggering beside our mom, who possessed nowhere near the size or strength to support him, they rushed forward.

They got Daddy back in bed and temporarily quieted Mom, but before they knew it, she had him up again, more determined than ever to make it to the parking lot.

By the time Michelle got there, Mom was convinced her own mother, who had died in 2000, was alive and being held hostage by the hospital staff.

When I arrived at their house at six, Mom was ranting about Michelle dumping her and Nana (Mom's mother) at the hospital, forcing her to take a taxi home.

I tried to explain what had actually happened, I never argued with my mother, not even as a teenager, but in that moment, it was incredibly important Mom understand that we—neither

Michelle nor I—would ever abandon her. Offering that comfort felt necessary, but she wouldn't

hear it.

Mom was so furious, she ordered me out. "You need to leave."

Pulling out a bit of my mother in me, I dug in. "Mom, the nurses had to call hospital security to

stop you from taking Daddy out of the hospital. Why would the nurses make that up? You were

trying to get Daddy out of the hospital and come home."

"I did no such thing!"

"But you did, and I know you were just tired, but—"

I could have pointed out the many flaws in her abandonment claims or Nana or locked hallways

but what was the point? I only wanted her to understand that she and Daddy were being taken

care of, but nothing is ever easy with Mom. Her temper runs hot and always has.

When she told me to leave, I had no idea how dark the foreshadowing of her final statement was.

"We'll be fine without you. We've managed this long, and we don't need your help."

Chapter Four

April 2017

> *Took my parents to the doctor today. Mom was in a loop and it went like this:*
> *Mom: Whose glasses are these?*
> *Alex: Those are yours.*
> *Mom: They're mine?*
> *Alex: Those are yours.*
> *Mom: They're mine?*
> *Alex: Yes, those are yours. (I didn't mind the repeated questions because I really needed*
>   *Mom to not notice Daddy was wearing her shirt.)*
> *We were almost done when...her eyes kind of squinted.*
> *Mom: Is that my shirt?!?!*
> *Alex: Whaa—? Nooo! Oh, don't be absurd! Daddy could never wear one of your shirts!*
>   *(Yeah. That's your favorite shirt, Mom, and might I say...he's wearing it well)*
> *Uncertain, she went along with it until we got into the car.*
> *Mom: Whose glasses are these?*
> *Daddy: Oh... [and he reaches over and puts them on!]*

I was mad at my mom. The details of exactly why are unimportant, but being forced to transition from repressing anger to understanding and accepting dementia made things a little more complicated but also beneficial.

Mom and me—we're good.

I had an awesome childhood. My sister and I giggle and snicker to this day over our harrowing experiences travelling around the world as kids because 1) we survived them, but also 2) we recognize how extraordinary our lives were. We were nearly accosted by a drunken Turk on a train from Russia to Finland. We nearly went down in a Tunisian airliner over the Mediterranean Sea. Then, there's the time we were forced to sleep on thousands of dead mountain moths (the result of a stupid lion and our father) in Kenya. We ran from KGB in the streets of Moscow and, as preteens, could successfully curse in six different languages. We learned to hold our own in Denmark lines where—though a very polite people by nature—it's first come, first serve. No lines.

In the 70s, while I was technically wearing roller skates, I marched in my first political rally in front of the White House, and we regularly hosted African military attachés in our home. I had breakfast with the famous U.S. ice hockey team (the players that inspired *Miracle on Ice*), lunch with Mohammed Ali, and dinner with Egyptian, Saudi, many African, and even British royalty. I sat on a curb with Elton John, and slipped into an elevator with Senator Ted Kennedy. I also learned, while running for my life through the orchards of a remote castle in southern France, that our faithful beagle/lab mix had no allegiance to me whatsoever when the hounds were released and we had to make it to the castle's kitchen before being mauled. When I hear the expression, *release the hounds,* I have a totally different perspective than most.

The point being, ours was not a normal upbringing and our memories are as wild as they are true. Throughout it all, however, our mother was not happy. Whether she was unhappy as a result of the constant travel that came with being a military wife or one who suffered from chronic depression, we will never know. One thing was certain, even as kids, we knew she was unsettled. When Daddy went off to Vietnam, she displayed behavior unbecoming of an officer's wife when Mom thought it prudent to invite a very popular band to our home for a party in the most inappropriate way. During the 70s, in particular, the unwritten rule was *if a military officer couldn't control his own woman, how could he control his troops?* But we were stationed in Honolulu, Hawaii, and Don Ho was a big name. Mom heard he and his band were coming to the big island, so she climbed on the roof of our home and spelled out an invite.

It worked.

I have zero memory of the event, but if the tales are anything to go by, apparently, the party was a doozy.

In the years that followed, Mom did not tow the good wife line. Rather, she went where her political and social conscious took her. Of this, I am most proud. Mom toted people to voting polls, gave the unemployed jobs and new ways to earn money and respect, and she always fought for the underdog, no matter how unpopular. But, with Daddy gone all the time and his job taking priority, she was also lonely. He loved Mom passionately and truly, but his country was his first love.

Mom got hit on a lot. So much so that it wasn't unusual for it to happen right in front of her children. I still remember standing in line at a restaurant when a man handed me a note to deliver to my mother. I remember feeling proud as I read: *You have the most beautiful brown eyes*. She did!

When I was in the fourth grade, we were assigned to a new post while our father finished up some military research. Mom used that time to travel to Oklahoma to finish her college degree. Just nine years old, I sensed something was not quite right with all the pictures of Mom lying out by a pool with fellow grad and undergrad students, most of whom were young men. But when the American Embassy was set ablaze in the Soviet Union and U.S. Navy Construction Forces (NCF) workers were brought in for repairs, Mom's friendship with one of the Seabees went beyond "not quite right."

Seabee is a term that comes from the initials CB, which stands for *construction battalion*, but for many, it also represents a pretty rough-and-tumble crowd known for heavy drinking and carousing.

The military officers' community is small, but life in an American Embassy overseas is even smaller and rumors run rampant.

ed my father's shame and my mother's

ssy's basement commissary. The ramp,

perfect skateboard ramp. Having recently

ding, I was feeling pretty sure of myself as

an women talking about my parents.

hed in my brain and, suffice to say, it was

of infidelity, political aspirations,

on a face-slapping clarity for me. I went

from being immature for my age to knowing way too much.

Mom reacted to the rumors by leaving the country with her Seabee friend, and Daddy responded

in kind by, most nights, drinking himself into a stupor.

Our Russian/KGB maid, Vera, took care of dinner preparations each night, but well after she left,

I was the one who put my father to bed, cleaned up the kitchen, and set his alarm for the next

day. The following mornings, Daddy would be long gone by the time I got up and moving, and I

was left wondering if he had any recollection of the night before, if he ever questioned how he'd

gotten to bed or who had set the alarm.

I drank, too, and at age thirteen, was quite the little bartender. Vodka was incredibly easy to

come by, and while the babushkas (older Russian women) scowled disapprovingly at my

purchases, I took full advantage.

Knowing what I do now, I imagine the KGB very much enjoyed my purchases as I fattened up

their intel file on Daddy. For this, I am both ashamed and sorry.

After another scandal surfaced, this time with a member from the U.S. hockey team, I felt as

though I was left with no other choice but pretending I had no idea what was going on. My shame and embarrassment were strong, but I couldn't decide whom I was most angry with—my

father for putting up with it or my mother for pulling us all down.

The next decade was more of the same.

Michelle's own curse was that she was never around to witness such humiliations. While I was

in Russia, she was in London. When we transferred to the U.S., she was at college. Ironically, for

those reasons, she was outwardly angry with our parents. It was her way of protecting me, of

apologizing to me, of making amends. But to what end? No matter how many times I told her

that these were not her mistakes and not her responsibilities, her pain and guilt were there.

I, on the other hand, never spoke of what I saw and heard. I buried it. Even as a teenager, I did

not argue, yell, or slam doors. I was, in all honesty, very happy with life. I went on to graduate

from college, marry, have children, and Michelle and I both earned positions on the first ever

U.S. women's bobsled team with Mom as our greatest cheerleader and supporter.

Mom was a fantastic grandmother and my children absolutely worshipped her! She was fun and

silly; she was whimsical and adoring. She gave prizes *and* surprises. What's not to love?

Following my bobsledding stint, I began a writing career and Mom was right there, supporting

me the whole way. She helped edit manuscripts and assisted with promotions. Admittedly, it

wasn't that hard to get published the first go-round because how many pregnant, national

champion female bobsledders were there in the world? Still, I had Mom to thank for much of

that.

The mother I adored as a young child was back, but while my relationship with our mother

flourished, Michelle's regressed.

Much of our teen and adult frustration with our parents stemmed from inattentiveness. More

aptly put, our parents were not parents. They were great stand-ins. They were well-meaning guardians, but actual parenting was never their strong suit. With Daddy saving the world, and

Mom looking for her next great cause between battles with her own anger and depression, it was

fortunate for them that Michelle and I were relatively well-behaved kids. I mean, ya know, minus

my drunken stupors, illegal pool hopping, and roaming the streets. Besides all that, I was great!

As a small child, Michelle fell and ruptured her spleen, but no one caught the fracture in her neck

brought on by the same fall. The following two decades, however, were filled with chronic

headaches and misery, leaving Michelle baffled that neither of her parents had picked up on her

varying, non-typical childhood medical issues. What normal kid downs entire bottles of aspirin

every month?

By her mid-twenties, she had developed ulcers from all the aspirin and Tylenol.

In her thirties, Michelle was T-boned at an intersection. The accident re-broke her neck, and no

amount of over-the-counter pill touched her pain. There was no mistaking the medical problem

this time, though. In just a few short years, Michelle developed a full-blown addiction to pain

medication that cost her everything—her job, her house, her car, her social life, her money.

My parents were not helping. They complained mightily yet supported Michelle's habit. They

enabled her so completely that it almost killed her. The twist was, the mistakes and

responsibilities that should have weighted my parents' shoulders down became hers, and when

she needed help most, when she needed tough love to come in and set things right, it was not

there. She didn't just stumble and fall…she crashed and burned.

Today, Michelle's guilt concerning the amount of money our parents spent on her nearly cripples

my bright, funny, sometimes silly, mostly sad, beautiful sister. She is awash with feelings of self-

reproach for something she had very little control over.

My frustration and rage with my parents rose.

It was while Michelle was living in Mom and Daddy's house, recovering physically and financially, that our attitudes regarding our parents flipped. Michelle adopted my *comme ci, comme ça* flair for life. Well, in all honesty, she was too impaired by medication to care. I, in turn, developed a new sense of protectiveness for my sister as well as my own growing family. For decades, our dad had been a functional alcoholic and slowly, though unintentionally—yet oddly deliberate—he turned our mom into one, too. It had only taken a few times of Mom, aka Mimom, having completely drunken conversations with her grandchildren, my children, for me to put a stop to it. Michelle, inebriated in her own way, was incapable of knowing or caring about what was going on. So, while the three of them lived together, outside the Beltway, I maintained a rule in my Texas household—no phone calls accepted from Mom or Daddy after 6 pm, central (my time). By 7 pm, eastern (their time), the odds that both parents were liquored to the gills were always excellent. The calls were unhealthy, as I was transported back to my pre-teen, teen, and young adult life listening to the slurred, inaudible conversations in which stories were repeated over and over. And nothing spelled *fun* like suffering through an inane forty-five-minute conversation only to discover the following day the person drudging you through that verbal misery had absolutely no memory of speaking to you in the first place. After surviving my late teens, keeping Friday-night vigil at the front door, waiting for Mom to return from a night of drinking with co-workers while Daddy was stationed at the Pentagon and travelling extensively throughout the African continent and Middle East, I wasn't about to be forced to reckon with certain behaviors again as an adult. I remembered far too well putting my drunken mother to bed after she had driven herself home.

Instead, I took on the role of church lady and berated my parents for drinking too much. It was, I'm sure, something they did not appreciate, but I was no longer interested in being drunk-dialed by my own parents. With my own children, I did not then and do not now drink or allow alcohol in my home.

It was another rule made perfectly clear to my parents, and soon enough they told me they had stopped drinking and were only buying non-alcoholic beer. While I never fully believed them, I hoped for more restraint.

Ours is a family steeped in addiction, from alcohol (mostly) to prescription drugs and marijuana to OCD, bipolar, and depression. My grandparents were alcoholics and extended family members have had serious addiction/medical issues. I don't pretend to understand it and it's certainly not fair, but for whatever reasons, the addictive genes seemed to have skipped me and settled quite comfortably on my parents and sister. For the sake of Michelle, I once told my parents, "You've got to knock this crap off!" But how is that supposed to translate to someone with an addiction?

It doesn't. Addiction is feverish in its wants and needs and does not go away easily.

With some effort, I convinced Michelle to move to Texas, but the road to recovery was hard. Every day was a new fight for Michelle, some better than others. Eventually, she won the battle but it left scars. She ran a full marathon with me, she got a job, she found a career in teaching— something she is very good at—made friends, and began making a home.

Together, we began to forgive our parents.

They were (and are) amazing human beings who helped more people than we could possibly count. They taught us about equality and empathy and charity. Racial slurs or derogatory language of any sort was never allowed in our home. They taught us how to treat others and that life was so much more than getting. Giving, we learned, was the key to true happiness.

Once, around 1974, while chauffeuring most of our soccer team in the family station wagon, there was an ongoing discussion of what we could all do for fun when a kid named Nikki suggested we go "nigger-knocking!"

Screeeech!

Mom slammed the brakes so hard that, as the station wagon slid to a stop, a squealing chorus of pre-teen girls (unbelted because it was the 70s) could be heard on both coasts as we smashed and mushed all over each other. Mom's head turned in such a way—it was a seated whirl—and her eyes were blazing. It was like the movie *Carrie*, and Mom was about to unleash holy terror on some poor soul. "Who said that?"

Hell almighty!

Every girl in the car pointed at Nikki.

Instinctively, Nikki understood—*She's whirling! She's whirling!*

To this day, I believe it is unlikely Nikki ever said that word again. While Daddy rescued nations and people from political coups, Mom rescued everyone and everything else, from ex-cons looking for new employment (that was how I scored my first "hot" piece of jewelry. Mom was perfectly mortified when she found out, but at eleven years old and in possession of stolen goods, I was so amped!) to poor children looking for a Christmas present. Mom even adopted an entire family for about ten years. She rescued animals and once unleashed her own reign of terror, using the media, on a homeowner's association after she discovered a board member had arranged for a friend's tree company to top trees just so the friend could profit at the expense of the HOA. Several trees died as a result launching Mom on a tree crusade. No matter how big or small (or tall) the cause, Mom was the voice of the people (and trees).

She was also uncharacteristically cool for a woman in her position. Specifically, as the wife of one of the highest-ranking U.S. Embassy diplomats.

Michelle and I grew up all too aware of the snobbery that comes with high-ranking officers. While we personally witnessed women getting a soldier or low-ranking officer in trouble for some minor offense, like not saluting her—which, by the way, we were taught a soldier should only salute another military brother/sister but not the spouse as s/he did nothing to warrant such respect—our mother never made such demands.

There's no better example of just how cool our mom was than the time we were in Tunisia, 1989. Michelle and I had flown out for Christmas and were promptly invited to an embassy party. It was the Who's Who of Embassy Row among many nations.

My grandmother, Nana, couldn't wait to inform me that the new staff sergeant's wife was attending the party, but many Americans, according to Nana, were concerned about this woman's behavior. Apparently, she had bleached blonde hair (gasp) and tattoos (double gasp)! Honestly, I was far more concerned about the Tunisians losing my luggage and, in doing so, forcing me to wear my grandmother's polyester pants. So not cool. Especially when the said blonde, tattooed, and yes, really inappropriately dressed wife of the staff sergeant approached Mom.

Cue the awkward silence.

She nodded at Mom, looked her up and down and said, "Your outfit is totally bitchin'."

Mouths dropped open.

I think the wife of the Japanese ambassador passed out.

In the diplomatic world, this could have gone south so quickly, and as I mentioned, we knew many women who would have seen to it that the staff sergeant was punished for such insubordination and uncouth behavior.

Instead, Mom looked down, ran her hands down the fabric, smoothing every hint of a wrinkle that dared show, then smiled at the woman. "Yes, bitchin'. Well, thank you."

Of course, by comparison, standing beside me in my polyester pantsuit, Mom was totally bitchin', but the point was how cool our mom was.

In a time when homosexuality was not at all accepted, our parents counseled, *to thine own self be true*. They supported others. They gave hope. They were progressive. It was the 60s and 70s, and Archie Bunker ruled the airwaves. Our parents, however, befriended people of every race, creed, color, sex, national origin, religion, sexual orientation, gender identity, disability, marital and socioeconomic status in a way that was genuine, honest, and open. They rocked. They really did. They just kind of sucked at being parents.

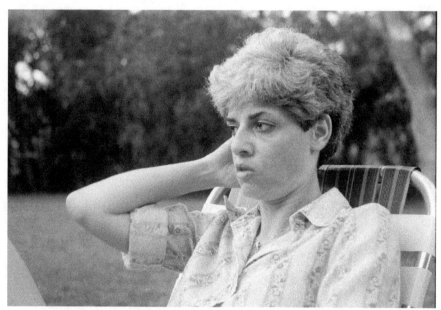

Candid Karen, in Dallas, during the late 1970s—no makeup, classic beauty

Chapter Five

July 2017

> *That moment when you walk into memory care and see the worried looks on staff's faces, and they're using walkie-talkies...*
> *Staff 1: Look behind all doors and under beds.*
> *Staff 2: We have! He's nowhere.*
> *Staff 1: Don't panic. We'll find him. We always do. Just don't panic.*
> *You know who they are talking about and...you feel an odd moment of pride.*

We have a marvelous family friend who was paralyzed in a freak bicycle accident. At the time of his accident, he was an athlete, powerfully built firefighter in Fort Worth, Texas, slated to be the next battalion chief of the department. It was a horrific event that left everyone stunned.

Afterward, he said, "No one plans on being paralyzed."

He's right! For that matter, I'm fairly certain Daddy never planned on doing a face-plant on his own kitchen floor and becoming permanently brain damaged. Who plans for such a thing?

I was sitting in church when Michelle called. My phone was on vibrate, as always, in case of an emergency, which seemed to be more often than not. Michelle and I lived every day awaiting the newest crisis. Mom lost her purse, didn't know where her wallet was, or was sure she had been robbed...or Daddy was hurt again.

Just a few weeks prior, he had driven himself to the ER, *again*. This time because he'd sliced open his thumb.

I braced myself. Sure enough, an unexpected text followed.

Aunt Elizabeth died last night.

I never saw that one coming.

Our Aunt Elizabeth, our father's baby sister, was a raging alcoholic, complicated by bipolar disease. She'd had countless seizures and while we all knew that alcohol would one day kill her, I was still shocked to learn she was gone at the young age of fifty-four.

Because she died in her home and there was a tremendous backlog for the coroner's office in the city of Dallas, it was several weeks before a proper autopsy was performed. For multiple reasons, the family decided to have her funeral to mid-January so that everyone could attend.

Thanksgiving and Christmas of 2015 flew by with almost comical scenarios starring our parents—who's on first, what's on second—still with the knowledge that Elizabeth's funeral awaited us.

We were invited to dinner where, supposedly, Daddy was grilling some of his mystery meat. The meat was tartare—it never even passed by a hot grill—the buns were burned, the vegetables were uncooked (not a huge deal but some really needed cooking), and we were all forced to sit on one side of the table, shoulder to shoulder (no one knows why), while we pretended to eat.

The best part was Michelle, the vegetarian, being served raw meat.

"Go ahead, Michelle," I urged, gleeful. "Try it!" It was my turn to exact more revenge on my sister for something she had done more than thirty years ago, in Central Asia. A place where meat was sparse.

Mostly, we ate regional vegetables, variations of breads, and pastries during our stay, but one night, we were served what looked like steak—my favorite.

But as I prepared to dig in, Michelle leaned close.

"That's elephant," she whispered.

What? I was horrified. I loved elephants. I couldn't eat an elephant! "Are you sure?"

As the daughters of a high-ranking attaché, we were often fed things which seemed horrifying to us, yet deemed cultural fare for our hosts. Each time, our father would shoot us a look—*the* look.

Our refusal to eat some variation of brain, liver, tongue, or eyeball of an animal we would have otherwise only seen in a zoo was considered an insult, and so, with extreme agony, we always picked up our forks and managed a few small bites.

Seeing the dread on my face at the very real possibility of being served elephant Michelle, my brilliant, protective older sister, took one for the team and ate both our elephants.

Later, when I'd learned the *steak* had been prepared just for us, I had been enraged. Compounding the insult of that night, Michelle went and turned vegetarian!

So, with my mother and father watching and giving my best impression of Daddy's "the look," I goaded Michelle on as she glared at me with a pained expression. "Go ahead. Try it. You'll like it." But when my son, Tommy, tried to raise his food to his mouth, I discreetly pushed his hand back toward his plate. "Don't eat that. You'll die."

We still giggle over the fact that my middle child, Katie, received a dog's squeaky toy for a gift, while many others got nothing because Mom forgot who was who.

The big un-funny was realizing Mom could no longer follow recipes she had been making for more than fifty years, like our grandmother's famous twenty-four-hour salad. It was a Powe tradition and Mom had mastered our Mumser's yummy marshmallow salad.

Operative word: had.

The head scratcher was my father thinking he could bring the ingredients for the twenty-four-hour salad out just minutes before dinner…for a recipe that takes, well, *twenty-four hours* to set.

Had we been paying more attention, we would have realized how disconnected our father was, but we were too distracted by Mom.

Thirty minutes into dinner, Mom wanted to go home. She used Colby as her reason.

We know now that the diseases of Alzheimer's and dementia were screaming in her ear.

She was desperate to make Daddy understand she had to leave right that minute, but he was on a roll.

"It's not about me, but it's the sixty-eight thousand who never came home." It was a Vietnam reference and his new catch phrase.

Michelle and I grew up in a home in which he never spoke of Vietnam. We knew no war stories, and it wasn't until we saw him speaking to hundreds of cadets at Texas A&M University that we learned he'd once had a gun pulled on him by a scared Iowa farm boy who didn't want to "take the hill" but just wanted to go home. We never fully appreciated the story of our father refusing to report the frightened young soldier, believing a private one-on-one conversation was better than a permanent reprimand.

Later, much later, we learned that it was stories like the Iowa farm boy that earned our father the greatest respect among his men.

By Thanksgiving of 2015, however, there were constant war references that no one understood. With so many of the family gathered, well-meaning loved ones tried to get Mom to stay. They cajoled and pleaded until she became very ugly.

Michelle and I were thoroughly embarrassed. We knew they didn't understand and only saw Mom misbehaving. In truth, we didn't understand it either.

As implausible as it sounds, the new year brought new hope, and we were feeling pretty good. Michelle had made a discovery concerning Daddy.

Almost daily, Michelle dropped by our parents' house on her way home from work and answered the phone because it was almost always ringing, but Daddy couldn't hear it and Mom could never find it.

On this particular day, the person on the other line identified herself as a nurse from Dr. Moody's office.

Michelle recognized the name and responded in kind.

We knew Daddy was seeing a doctor regarding neurological issues but had few details beyond what we'd learned when we'd reached out to two of our father's best friends, Colonels Baisden and Nicholas—white spots had been found on Daddy's brain scan—but even the colonels' knowledge was limited on how extensive the issue was or how secretive our father had become.

Only a few months prior, Daddy had made a trip back to Washington D.C., on his own, for a Moscow Embassy reunion. Most military intelligence officers retired in the D.C. area, and every few years, the American crew tried to get together.

When he landed, he rented a car, almost immediately got lost, and then began calling Mom for help.

Mom couldn't even turn the computer on, and so she called me for guidance.

I immediately called Daddy, but he was so flustered he couldn't concentrate on what I was saying and ended our call.

Eventually, he found his way and had a pleasant reunion, but we were a bundle of nerves back in Texas the entire time he was gone. Although he had done it for years and years, the thought of him driving in D.C. traffic was terrifying. During his trip, he shared two things with a few former colleagues. First, he and Mom were definitely moving back to D.C. in the spring, and second, he needed to have a minor procedure done regarding some neurological issues.

When he landed in Dallas, he called Mom. His car had been stolen.

Right on cue, Mom called me in a panic. She needed me to call Daddy because his car was stolen, all his belongings were stolen, and he was stranded.

What?! I called Daddy who instantly picked up. "What's up?" I was playing it cool and hoping Mom was wrong.

"Well, my car has been stolen," he said.

"But you weren't robbed or anything?" After listening to Mom's version, I had visions of him being carjacked.

"No! I came back to the spot where I parked my car and—"

Oh. "Well, maybe you're just in the wrong spot," I suggested, and boy, did he get mad! I tried to make a joke of it, tell him how many times I wandered an airport parking lot, with no idea where I had left my car, but he was insistent his had been stolen.

He said he was taking a taxi home and would deal with the car theft later. I tried to talk him into letting me pick him up, but he was determined to take a taxi home for prideful reasons only.

Another hundred-dollar taxi ride. So, I lied. I said I was going into Dallas to drop off a package and would literally be mere minutes from his location.

When he finally relented, I called the airport police and laid it out—my father, who is suffering from early-onset dementia, believes his car has been stolen from the airport parking lot, but I guarantee it is still there.

Sure enough, after driving Daddy around for the better part of an hour, an officer with the airport police department found his car.

Nothing was ever mentioned about the incident again, but Michelle and I began having serious discussions about how much longer Daddy should be allowed to drive.

At the time, telling your father he should no longer drive was a terrible position to be in. His car was such a large part of his independence. How could we possibly take the keys away?

But...Lady Luck was with us, at last!

Michelle's conversation with Dr. Moody's nurse yielded interesting information. Apparently, Daddy had hydrocephalus (aka *water on the brain*). It causes confusion, inability to recall words, imbalance, and several other symptoms we immediately identified with Daddy's current medical concerns.

I imagined similar conversations occurring in other homes around the nation—families discovering their father had water on the brain. Shock. Instant worry. Fear. But Michelle and I were elated.

It explained so much.

No. Wait. This explains everything! So...why wouldn't he tell us that? Never mind. It doesn't matter. This is seriously good news. He doesn't have dementia. He's going to be okay. High fives!

Water on the brain was reversible, right? A shunt in the base of his skull would help relieve the water off his brain then he would be back to his brilliant self. He would finish that military intelligence book he was going to write.

While we were certainly concerned about the procedure itself and understood there were no guarantees, we knew our dad. He's a tough old soldier, and this was going to make a huge difference. After all, we learned Daddy had already attempted the procedure once before but had been turned away when the hospital had realized Daddy came alone. Despite explaining how the procedure would work—a family member must be present and he wasn't allowed to drive for two weeks afterward—Marc Powe had shown up like it was a dental cleaning.

Michelle told the nurse there was an excellent chance Daddy never really heard them since he was pretty much deaf and rarely adjusted his hearing aids to a proper setting.

That was when the nurse said they had also explained it all to Mom.

"Yeah. Well, our mom has Alzheimer's."

Again, as sad as that information was to say, we counted it as another score for our team. The more people who understood Mom's medical situation, the better we could care for both parents. And again, knowing Daddy's problems could be relieved was a huge burden lifted from our shoulders. Things—positive things—were set in motion.

Operation Daddy-Just-Needs-A-Shunt was a go after Daddy's preoperative appointment, and he was given strict instructions that he could not drive.

Awesome. I will be his chauffeur.

What was not so awesome was, despite knowing exactly where we were going, Daddy insisted on bringing his GPS.

When I pulled up to the house, he was already waiting outside, ball cap pulled low over his forehead and shoulders stooped in intense concentration, punching in the address on his GPS. As he got into the car I let him know we didn't need it.

"I turned on the GPS so it can safely guide us there," he said.

Okay. He probably didn't hear me. "OH, WE DON'T NEED THAT, DADDY!"

The ever-so-helpful GPS made its techno-voiced announcement—*You have arrived at your location.*

Sigh. I pulled away from the curb and away we went.

I had gotten Daddy a coffee and a copy a of the *New York Times* from Starbucks beforehand, so he was momentarily distracted and happy as he read every headline, out loud.

Turn right in thirty feet.

"SO, I REALLY DO KNOW WHERE WE ARE GOING—"

Turn right at the next—

Daddy read on while I suggested that maybe he had put his home address as the final destination because it sounded as though the damned GPS was just trying to turn us around.

Rerouting.

"DADDY! I DON'T THINK THAT THING IS WORKING!"

At the next intersection, take Butler Road.

"BECAUSE IT JUST SEEMS LIKE IT'S—"

Rerouting.

"DADDY! THIS IS GOING TO BE A LONG-ASS TRIP IF WE KEEP REROUTING!"

At the next intersection, make a U-turn.

"SERIOUSLY, DADDY! I THINK THAT THING IS—"

Rerouting.

And so it went for another thirty miles through early morning Dallas traffic.

When we reached the parking garage, Daddy finally turned off the GPS.

I'm pretty sure that marked the moment my carpel tunnel developed, as I was gripping the steering wheel so hard my fingers were tingling. I made a mental note to "accidentally" stomp the crap out of the GPS system when he wasn't looking.

We headed for the pre-op area, got a clipboard for patient information and, while I noted a somewhat startled expression on the part of the nurse at the admittance desk, I was too busy thinking, "rerouting…rerouting…rerouting…" and steered us toward two seats in the lobby.

Daddy stuffed the cap he'd removed as we had entered off to the side and sat to my left.

That was the first time that I actually saw the right side of his face. "Daddy!" I was horrified.

How did I miss this?

He looked up. "Hmm?"

"What happened to your face?" Stunned, I replayed the morning in my head.

His head had been down when he'd approached the car. Then, he had sat in the passenger seat,

so I'd never noticed his glasses were askew or the rims were cracked. I hadn't seen the black eye,

the cut on his ear and jawline, and the massive bruising all down the right side of his face.

"I don't know," he said, a little too slowly, as he lightly touched his face.

"You don't know?" I, of course, said that a little too loudly, and other people turned to look at us

and gaped at Daddy's face.

He shrugged. "I don't know."

"When did that happen?"

"Don't know." Another shrug.

"Did you trip?"

"Don't know."

Even now, all this time later, I recall looking across the small sitting area and locking eyes with

another woman openly staring. I remember her making a *sorry* expression and shrugging.

Somehow, we both sensed I probably stood a better chance at learning what happened to my

father from her, a stranger, than my own dad.

I hadn't noticed and silently berated myself. I had been so distracted by that infernal GPS system

and Daddy's deafness that I had not detected he was more off than usual. He had been content

with his coffee and paper.

The bruising on his face was massive, and I had to know. "Did it happen while you were walking

Colby?"

But he only shrugged again and again as I pressed.

At last, he unknowingly offered up a clue when he mentioned it was lucky he'd found his

glasses.

Ah.

He mentioned finding them on his kitchen floor, and the more we talked, the more we concluded

he must have fallen in the kitchen.

"I guess so." And one final shrug, for good measure.

Until this point, every time Michelle or I had pressed for any legal standing in our parents'

affairs, they'd shut us down. When we had tried to get on the Health Insurance and

Accountability Act or HIPPA form, allowing medical professionals to share information with us,

Mom had put a stop to that immediately, saying we were being intrusive and "trying to take

control." Even when I'd attempted to appeal to Mom's love for her husband by saying, "But

something is going on with Daddy. We just want to be sure he is okay," she had shut me down.

Mom had made sure we had no standing whatsoever. Her comeback line had always lingered

around the *pure hateful* end of the spectrum. "Don't worry. You'll be well taken care of in the

will."

What the hell?

Daddy's name was called to have his blood work done, and he rose.

The nurse at the Dallas Methodist Hospital winced when she saw his face.

As Daddy headed back, I was shooting texts to Michelle, my husband Robb, and a friend who's a

nurse of the picture I'd managed to take just before the nurse had come out.

Michelle's reply was immediate. *What happened?*

But my friend's response was more helpful. *You need to have him checked out. Probable*

concussion.

I decided to creep into the lab where they were doing blood work and mention his accident. We were in a hospital, after all. Why not have him checked out while we were there?

Before I could make it to the lab, however, I ran into the nurse who had collected Daddy already on her way back out to find me.

She asked if he was always incoherent.

Well, yes and no. I explained what I knew, both with the current accident but during the last year.

"Do you have medical power of attorney?" she asked.

I told her 'no' and that my parents had been very resistant, despite my mother's Alzheimer's and Daddy's … whatever he had going on. She gave me a look. "Oh, that's going to change."

True statement: Nurses make things happen. Nurses are the true caregivers, and doctors are just decoration. Nurses run the medical field and rule supreme!

She convinced Daddy to sign over medical power of attorney to me right there on the spot.

As a note of clarification, this medical power of attorney has nothing to do with the fight we would soon have for an actual full power-of-attorney status. I realize now the medical power of attorney was both easy and a mere warm-up for what was to come.

Two days later, we were sitting at Aunt Elizabeth's funeral. It was a tough go, listening to the Powe siblings—Uncle Stephen, Uncle Chris, and Aunt Diana—cry softly as we put their baby sister to rest. Their pain was palpable.

From Daddy, however, it felt like static electricity. There was this kind of numb-ish but very sad vibration coming from him. Nothing more.

His face looked far worse as the bruising had begun to change color and the blood had drained from the initial point of contact on the top right side of his forehead. He looked like he had been hit with a bat. He had also refused to see any other doctors while we were at the hospital, so we could only speculate whether or not he was concussed.

Stubborn as a fool, he had driven himself to the funeral and, of course, Mom hadn't attended since she couldn't leave Colby alone that long.

None of us argued. After all, there was going to be a small family reunion, the kind only funerals bring about, at our parents' house later that evening.

I cannot comment about the others, but I noticed that Daddy was drinking heavily and asked Michelle if that wasn't an even worse idea than usual. It was hard to know if it was the alcohol, grief, or a concussion spurring so many inappropriate and/or confused comments on Daddy's part.

One day later, approximately thirty hours after laying Aunt Elizabeth to rest, after everyone had returned to their homes and perspective lives, Daddy pulled another header on the ceramic-tiled floor. This time, he didn't get up.

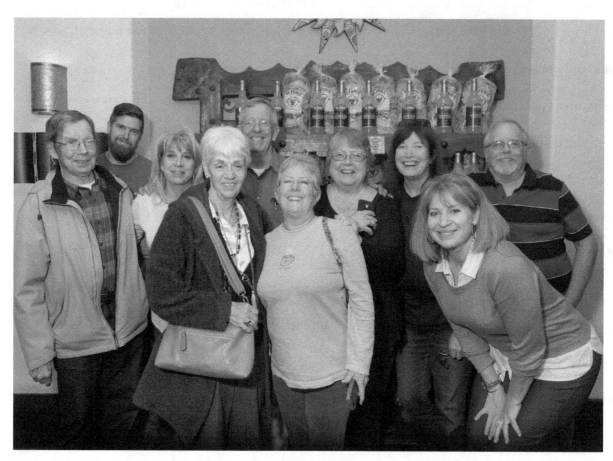

Following the funeral of Aunt Elizabeth, this is the last shot we have of a Powe gathering: Far left is Marc Powe, John Powe (cousin), Michelle (yellow sweater), Karen (in front), Stephen Powe (uncle), Susan Orr (cousin), Sandy Powe (aunt), Diana Powe (aunt), Chris Powe (uncle), and the author, Alexandra Allred (front right).

*Note about the turquoise bag Mom is holding. THAT is the infamous lost/found, lost/found, lost/found purse.

Chapter Six

FACEBOOK: August 2017

> *Alex: [speaking with the VA's Release of Information Department] ...all I need is information about who my father was seeing prior to his fall.*
> *ROI Dept: We can't tell you that.*
> *Alex: But, I have medical Power of Attorney.*
> *ROI Dept: We don't have record of that.*
> *Alex: Okay, but I do. I can bring it—*
> *ROI Dept: You'll have to bring that to whoever was seeing him.*
> *Alex: Ah, yes. Excellent point. So, who was that?*
> *ROI Dept: We can't tell you that.*
> *Alex: But you are the Release of Information.*
> *ROI Dept: Yes, ma'am.*
> *Alex: [seconds tick away] But you won't release that information?*
> *ROI Dept: No, ma'am.*
> *Alex: Because you're the Release of Information...*
> *ROI Dept: Yes, ma'am.*
> *Alex: Ah.*

My phone was vibrating by 6 o'clock the next morning. It was Michelle.

Foregoing any proper greeting when I answered, she was all business. "Daddy fell and I'm going to the hospital now. Can you go to the house to get Mom? She's pretty shook up."

As best as we could piece together, Mom found Daddy on the floor sometime between midnight and 6 am. With Alzheimer's, day and night are often confused, but Mom said that she had woken up next to him and realized she needed to call for help. We found her pillow on the kitchen floor, so we believe she found him, was unable to rouse him, and she simply lay down on the tile floor beside him.

When she awoke, new light brought better clarity and that was when she called 911, which was great, but the clarity wasn't all-inclusive. She could not remember his name.

The EMTs brought Daddy in as a John Doe, and for a brief and scary time, Michelle was unable to find our father in the hospital. Worse, she actually thought he died, and the staff just didn't want to tell her.

Meanwhile, I arrived in time to find Mom "walking" Colby around the coffee table in the living room.

She made two more circles with the poor dog, and I really started pushing our need to go.

"I have to walk Colby."

Another circle.

"Okay, Mom, but now we really need to go. Daddy needs us."

"I have to walk Colby. When I get back from the walk then we can go." She circled again. And again.

I stepped forward and gently pulled the leash from her hand.

She looked confused and then horrified, as though Colby would break free and run wild in whatever pasture or far away land she imagined us to be in, and I assured her.

"He's good. Colby is walked. Now Daddy needs us."

Another ten minutes passed as Mom compulsively packed a bag for the trip. It made no sense to witness, but appeared perfectly logical to Mom. She packed socks, some straws, and a spoon.

She got a Nancy Drew book, some letters and paper, and a bunch of paperclips.

When I tried to urge her on, yet again, she got upset.

"I know, honey! But I can't go empty-handed!"

What happened next is still a bit of a blur due to the heaviness in my head and heart, but I do recall knowing well before the others did. I don't say that in a braggadocio manner but rather one of sorrow. I was fully aware of something the others did not want to know. Memories flooded my mind as I stood over Daddy's gurney, staring down at this heavily bruised man, his face now battered just as badly on the opposite side, and I knew. He was out cold, snoring. He was completely shit-faced.

But Michelle was his champion. She wanted to know how much the hydrocephalous factored into his fall. She wanted to know if the concussion (we were sure he'd had one) from his first fall had not caused the newest assault to his brain. She wanted his heart monitor assessed. She wanted to make sure this wasn't something to do with those white spots on his brain that Daddy had discussed with other people.

And while she rattled off every medication the man had ever taken or even thought about taking, I just watched the slow, steady breathing of my father and I knew.

Michelle was adamant. She knew in her heart, his fall was because he had not yet been treated for the hydrocephalus and just as soon as he had this procedure, he was going to be right again. He would be his old self again. He would be okay. She wasn't going to listen to me suggesting anything otherwise.

I tried not to sigh out loud. I tried not to sound defensive in any way. "There's broken glass on the kitchen floor, and it's all sticky from the alcohol. He was drinking, Michelle."

She acknowledged only that the ambulance drivers had mentioned smelling alcohol when they'd brought our father in. She acknowledged it only because that bit of information had already been relayed to various hospital staff.

But when the attending nurse returned with Daddy's blood work results, not even Michelle could deny the awful truth. His blood was three and half times the legal limit. Given his age and size, the nurse just shook her head. "I don't even know how he's still alive."

Judas Priest.

This was just the first of many medical blunders that made us realize how often guessing was standard medical procedure.

The next week was beyond awful. No one should watch a loved one go through what we watched our father endure.

It started out with the doctor performing the hydrocephalus procedure calling it off. Michelle was crushed, but the doctor did not mince words. Daddy was an alcoholic. The long-term damage done to his brain was yet to be determined. And as an added bonus, the doctor opted to share a story about his aunt who had gone through something very similar and was dead within six months.

How do you respond to something like that?

I just stared at him.

Initially, it appeared the doctor might be wrong. Daddy woke up. He was talking, reading the paper out loud, being social, and he was eager to leave the hospital.

As the days wore on, however, he slipped—not a little but a lot. His speech slurred, his agitation grew, and his balance worsened. So much so that he required an around-the-clock sitter as he seemed hell-bent on climbing out of his bed at every opportunity. Never mind that he couldn't walk, much less stand, he was determined to put on his jeans and leave the hospital.

Before our very eyes, his personality changed. His physical being and abilities changed.

And though we had worked with, spoken to, and asked questions of so many doctors, it ended up being one of my own gym students—a speech and language specialist—who nailed it after she heard about Daddy's falls, hitting first his right side and then his left. "Oh, wow! He hit both speech and personality."

The days turned into weeks, and we watched with dismay as our brilliant father, with his genius IQ, astounding vocabulary, and vast capacity to grasp and hold information, began babbling about nonsensical things. More often than not, however, he was simply polite. He thanked everyone, patted hands, and even kissed a few heads when nurses checked his vitals. Other times, however, it was a full-out wrestling match to keep him still.

"He's small," people commented, "but very strong."

Boy howdy!

And determined.

Every step of the way was complicated by Mom, which was only compounded by the fact that just moving with her was painful.

You have to understand, I move at the speed of light. I'm always on the go, with fifteen things happening at once. It's the reason no one volunteers to go grocery shopping with me. For me, shopping is an Olympic event.

Now, I am being forced to walk through parking lots and hospital corridors with a woman who— I swear—is doing it on purpose. A person simply cannot *accidentally* walk that slowly! That has to be on purpose. *Gawd. Mom. Please!*

Sometimes I walked backward, urging her forward. Other times I pointed things out. "Look, Mom. That caterpillar just walked by, and *he's waving!* All fifty of his left hands!" But I couldn't truly be mad. She was a mess.

Our lives were suddenly all about getting Mom to and from seeing Daddy in the hospital while still juggling our jobs, lives, and social/family responsibilities. If we weren't at the hospital, she wanted to go to the hospital, and if we were at the hospital, she wanted to go home.

If I could have gone back in time, I would have pressed Daddy to understand that, by allowing Mom to hole up in her house twenty years ago, he was only exacerbating Mom's confusion. Mom always sought refuge in her home and all the traveling back and forth was making her more confused than ever. But…her needs were insatiable, and it was our responsibility to meet them, period.

The reality was…we didn't. Not successfully, anyway.

To my mighty sadness, I had to give up my training classes at work while Michelle was reprimanded multiple times at her own job, and everything else fell to the wayside. But, again, the needs of our mother…

We drove back and forth and back and forth. We spent hours in Daddy's room only to return home and have her say, "Well, at some point today I would like to go see your father." She didn't remember we had just spent six hours with him, and there was no convincing her otherwise. She couldn't remember which doctors visited Daddy and was certain everyone was neglecting him. Regardless of pain, lack of speed, mounting confusion, Mom was determined to be by Daddy's side, whether she remembered it or not, and the one thing they accomplished together, in spectacular form, was declining in rapid succession.

Doctors tried to speak to Daddy while he was still able to talk. They asked him if he knew what time it was or what day or month it was; who the president was or when his birthday was, and of course, more often than not, Daddy could not say.

One day, as we drove home from the hospital, Mom asked, "Well, what did the man say?"

"What man?"

"The man who didn't know who the president was."

"Mom, that was Daddy."

"Don't be ridiculous! Your father knows who the president is."

When I reminded her that he had a head injury and was not of sound mind, she got mad.

"Well, how was I supposed to know that?" She accused me of cutting her out of the loop. Even though she was always present when we spoke to nurses and doctors about Daddy's condition and care, and even though Mom was there when Daddy fell, she insisted she knew nothing of what was happening.

It was on just such an occasion, yet another return trip from the hospital, when I was accused of withholding information about her husband, that I made yet another of many blunders. I said, "You just don't remember."

Ladies and gentlemen, this is exactly how *not* to handle a person with Alzheimer's. Don't do that.

During the first few weeks, we still had hope Daddy would return to his old self or close to it. Even after several doctors cautioned us that he wouldn't be allowed to drive for at least six months, we didn't think much about it.

For a person with Alzheimer's, however, future guidelines don't compute.

So, when I said, "Of course, he won't be able to drive for six months, but we'll get that covered," I was trying to be positive.

What Mom heard was that I was taking away their independence. She was furious. She was going to get a lawyer. She was going to sue Michelle and me. We had no right to dictate their lives, and she railed about learning to drive so she could take herself to and fro and no longer need us. Everyday there seemed to be some new argument from Mom—we were neglecting her needs or invading her privacy, sometimes both.

What was really happening was Michelle and I were getting very sick. Between all the germs

undoubtedly picked up in the hospital, the constant trips back and forth to Dallas, and the lack of

sleep, our parents were slowly—however unwittingly—destroying us. Both of us picked up a

hacking, lung-rattling cough, fever, and exhaustion…but Mom *had* to see her husband.

As Mom and I, once again, approached Daddy's room and heard beeping, we knew. At least, I

knew. He was out of bed, again.

The hospital kept restraints on my father, which was necessary but hard to see. Yet Marc, ever

the military dog, was able to rip them off and climb—or *attempt* to climb out of bed. It didn't

matter that he could not walk. He was determined to escape.

As we walked in, we found him in a tussle with one of the nurses.

I stepped in and helped her wrestle him back down. And no sooner than we got him settled, Mom

started.

"Where's my purse? Did I forget my purse? Have you seen my purse?"

Many times, I pointed out her purse to her and each time it brought her pleasant resolve.

"Oh!" Then, she noticed a monitor hanging over Daddy's bed, near his head, and noted that it

had a *press exit* button on the screen. For whatever reason, she felt the need to press it.

This is just one example of how our lives were going with Mom and Daddy during this time:

"No, Daddy! You can't stand up"

"Mom, your purse is right here. Don't touch that button."

"Daddy, why are you getting up?"

"It's right here, Mom. Yeah. No. Don't touch that."

"Daddy, you need to stay in bed."

"It's here. It's right here. I have your purse."

"Daddy, stay still."

"Nope. That would be a big no-no. Don't touch that."

"Rrrrrrright here. The purse is here."

"I don't think they want you to touch that button."

"Daddy! You can*not* stand up!"

"Yeah, I have it. I have your purse."

"I know it says press exit but they don't really mean it."

"Daddy, Dr. Moody said you have to stay in bed."

"Mom! It is right here."

"If you touch that button your hand will blow off."

"Daddy! It is *illegal* to stand up. It is against the law."

And then finally, "I have no idea where your purse is. Go ahead—push it!"

When the nurse walked in I said (very sweetly), "Hey, you know when, on the news, we see how a wild bear walks into a suburban neighborhood and he's scared and confused so we just get out the tranq guns and shoot him?"

"Yes."

"Why don't we just shoot my parents?"

Blank stare.

"I'll pull the trigger."

Continued blank stare.

Mom and Daddy weren't the only ones losing their minds. We were, too. Though Michelle and I found ways to keep ourselves entertained, Daddy's prognosis was bleak. The staff didn't much like him always trying to escape and Mom's utter confusion was draining. She asked the same questions again and again and again and again, and sometimes in such rapid succession we were baffled that she couldn't remember she had just asked that same questions seven times in a row in less than two minutes.

I began answering differently just to amuse myself.

Mom: [looks around the car as we head toward the hospital to see Daddy] I don't have my…purse. I need my purse.

Alex: You don't need your purse.

Mom: I don't? Why don't I? I need my ID.

Alex: You don't need your ID.

Mom: I don't? How will I get into the hospital to see Daddy?

Alex: They don't ask for your ID. We can just walk in.

Mom: Are you sure?

Alex: Positive. We've done it a bunch of times.

Not three minutes later, we repeated the same conversation.

Another two minutes pass, and the exact—to the word—conversation again.

Round four and…honestly, it's a long drive to the hospital:

Mom: [looks around the car as we head toward the hospital to see Daddy] I don't have my…purse. I need my purse.

Alex: You don't need your purse.

Mom: I don't? Why don't I? I need my ID.

Alex: You don't need your ID.

Mom: I don't? How will I get into the hospital to see Daddy?

Alex: They know us on sight and just wave us in.

Mom: They do? I don't remember that.

Alex: It's because we tip them excessively.

Mom: We do?

As we pulled into the hospital and after having had the conversation no less than eight times, my answers were becoming so fanciful that I began believing she remembered and was now just messing with my head.

Mom: [looks around the car as we head toward the hospital to see Daddy] I don't have my…purse. I need my purse.

Alex: You don't need your purse.

Mom: I don't? Why don't I? I need my ID.

Alex: You don't need your ID.

Mom: I don't? How will I get into the hospital to see Daddy?

Alex: After Daddy took out the KGB guy disguised as a nurse, they moved Daddy to the covert-operations wing of the hospital. We have top clearance. Of course, they have our eyeballs scanned and fingerprints, so no matter what we touch or look at, the security team will be alerted. In fact, they are watching us right now. This security team is top-notch.

Mom: [staring at me] Are you sure?

Alex: See that guy right there? [I wave at a random man walking past our car.]

Somewhat confused, but obliging, he waves back.

Alex: He's a spy guard. He's getting off duty now. His name is Alberto.

That was the same day I got home and found a book in the mail that I had apparently ordered—

The 36-Hour Day: A Family Guide to Caring for People Who Have Alzheimer's Disease,

Related Dementias, and Memory Loss by Nancy Mace and Peter Rabins. It's an incredible

resource but…holy shit, I had no memory of ordering this book. *Oh, man. I have dementia!*

Almost two weeks later, my friend, Mark Larkin, called to see if I'd received the book.

TIP: Here's what you don't do when you have a friend who has two parents with varying forms

of dementia: You don't order her a book, not tell her about it, and then let her go many, *many*

days wondering when she ordered a book about her oncoming dementia.

My mental state aside, I was beginning to wonder about my mother's sense of humor as I

watched Mom cut up a slice of pizza with garden scissors from the garage then have a long

conversation with me about grant writing for the National School Board Association.

I called Michelle into the room in whispered tones. "I think Mom's just screwin' with us! She's

not really demented. She knows what she's doing and she's torturing us for all the crap we pulled

as kids!"

If only.

Another night at the hospital, I realized we spent more time on Mom than Daddy. We were going

through the horrible motions, but nothing about what we did was for Daddy. We were appeasing

Mom, enduring Mom…handling Mom. We weren't talking to or working with Daddy at all. He

was just a zombie residing in the same space.

After work one early morning, I bought an interactive toy barn that required different windows

and doors to be opened. I knew it was babyish, and it was hard to buy something so childish, but

I also wanted to keep his curious mind occupied and give Daddy something to do with his hands.

In working with my special needs students, I knew how important it was to spur on cognitive thinking, keep him curious and motivated, and at this point, he had disassembled the arm to his chair, and days before, when we had wheeled Daddy toward the window, he'd pointed and said, "Crape myrtle" and "House."

I showed him pictures of the Chad helicopter he had apprehended from drug lords in the Chadian desert, and he said, "Machine," and "Ho, boy!"

Yes! He was remembering!

And when I told the story of Daddy securing money from the Pentagon to retrieve the downed helicopter before the Soviets got to it to one of our favorite nurses, Anthony, I picked up a copy of *Billion Dollar Spy* and flipped it open to the picture of the American Embassy and asked, "What's this?"

At first, Daddy said nothing but he looked at it.

The third time I asked, he said, "Embassy."

Oh, heck yeah, it is!

We were on a roll, and I wasn't about to let it slip past unnoticed. I pulled out the toy and opened the various latches and locks.

At first, he had zero interest, and I feared he felt I was patronizing him.

What was funny was each nurse who came in began to play with it, recognizing the value of the toy but—let's get real—they also just liked playing with all the latches.

Tony, another nurse, opened a barn door that revealed a cow and, to our happy surprise, Daddy said loudly, "Moo!"

We laughed and, Daddy was delighted.

He grinned and opened another door. There was a pig. "Oink!"

It wasn't just a moment for me but for Tony as well. How many times had the nurses and doctors remarked that Daddy was an exceptionally intelligent man, that they saw how he was suffering, that he wanted to know, he wanted to think, he wanted to speak and engage but simply could not? Here was this guy, one of the Pentagon's more brilliant minds, a war hero, a military intelligence expert, having done things we still don't and can't ever know about, and we were thrilled with his "moo" and "oink."

So, when he looked at the chicken, I knew I had to challenge him. I knew I had to, in some way, be a smart ass—*his* smart ass—and let him know I wasn't patronizing him, that I knew he was still in there somewhere.

Tony opened the next little window.

Daddy saw the chicken and said, "Cluck."

"Cluck? Who the hell says *cluck*? Daddy, you're not doing this right!" My heart was in my throat as I waited.

And he laughed.

Yeah. He knew. Chickens don't say cluck. *They say*, brawk. *Everyone knows that.*

While we discussed the finer nuances of animal noises, Mom was only mildly amused. She was lost.

When she wasn't lost, she was anxious. The moment our father moved, she was all over me or Michelle. "Michelle! Michelle! He's trying to get up," or "He's moving. He's—" She fussed over him but was also afraid of him. She knew she could not physically handle him, but she monitored every movement.

Their entire marriage had been one of control and if she had thrown enough of a fit, she had always gotten her way.

Suddenly, none of that worked or mattered to her husband, and she didn't know how to handle it.

She also learned that there was no point in walking with Daddy. She stayed behind when I took

him for little excursions because, much to the distress and disapproval of the nursing staff,

Daddy and I played Olympic Bobsled Trials!

Like me, Marc Powe had always moved quickly.

He never sat still, and so I knew he would appreciate flying through the hallways of the hospital

on his gurney like he was in a bobsled and, as it happened, I was really good at pushing

bobsleds...

Apparently, "somebody could get hurt," so I only ran short bursts of bob runs when no one was

looking, hung a hard left, and dead ended at the hallway where a large bay window allowed us to

look out onto Dallas' Bishop Avenue.

At the window, Daddy read signs of the local shops down below and we applauded his efforts.

It was two weeks after the fall and I sent out an email to friends and family letting them know

words are coming back, that he was reading out loud, and that he was funny. He was finding his

feet again too. He couldn't walk, but he could stand.

One day he decided he was going to take himself to the bathroom which, while awesome, could

not happen. It was too dangerous.

I told him we needed to call for a nurse.

He gave me a super defiant look.

"Daddy! I work out every day. If you want to throw down, we can do it right here, but you're not

winning."

While he was not amused, I knew he heard me. And he believed me. I was his kid, after all.

Like I'd told everyone in my email, we had a long, long way to go, but there were signs of improvement…and we had hope. Cluck.

Chapter Seven

I told Tommy to watch his grandfather.
Alex: Just make sure he doesn't pull the fire alarm. He's not fast but he's determined.
And Tommy chuckled. His grandfather is an old man with head trauma. How fast can he—
Fire alarm: Wwa-wwa-wwa-wwa!
Alex: Tommy! You let him pull the alarm?
Tommy: I didn't let him! He's got super powers or something!

Progressive diseases suck. That's one of the big takeaways here. Because you can go through therapy, rehab, there can be prayers and love, and all kinds of positive interaction, but progressive diseases easily take over and command the train. The ride is all about fighting for control of the engineer's cap. Then, at some point, the remainder of the trips is about finding a comfortable window seat so you can just appreciate the scenery.

After more than a month in the hospital, the staff was more than ready to see the ambulance carry our father to Ennis Care Center.

They are one of the very few facilities that will work with the VA and Medicare. To date, it is truly one of the best experiences we've had. While the building is rundown, by their own admission, the staff is top notch. I hope for the entire Ellis County community that funds can be appropriated for a new building to match the professionalism and kindness we received while there.

But our stay lasted no more than three weeks before we moved our father again due to geographical reasons for our mother. It took as much as two hours in Dallas traffic if there was an accident. Ennis Care was about an hour away in total, but Mom was incapable of understanding time.

Almost two months had come and gone, and Mom's Alzheimer's was reaching a new level. She

was more anxious than ever before and she desperately, desperately, *desperately* needed her

husband to come back to her. Her solution was to hover. She fussed, flitted, and moved around

him like a little hummingbird.

In response, he shoved her.

The physical pain was minor. She was more shocked than anything. But never was she more

emotionally injured.

Marc Powe worshipped her. Hers had always been the final word. Her wish had been his

command. He had endured more heartache and betrayal from this woman than any man should,

but he loved her so deeply that he had blamed himself for her indiscretions.

Now, he was pushing her away, and she couldn't understand why.

The more Michelle and I arranged for Mom to see Daddy, the more she asked for more. She

needed to see us more. She needed to see Daddy more. She needed everything…more.

We were beyond exhausted and, for the first time, I saw frustration and resentment creeping into

Michelle's psyche.

For Mom's sake, for convenience, to empower her in what little way we could, and to give

ourselves some rest, Michelle and I agreed to pay a little extra money and move Daddy closer to

home.

But it was a hard move. The new staff wasn't as accommodating. They did not want to put forth

the kind of effort that was required of our father. And so, they didn't. They just didn't.

Michelle and I now fancy ourselves pseudo-experts in memory- and senior-care facilities. We

understand there is no such place as "perfect" because there are simply too many moving parts to

Alzheimer's/dementia/Parkinson's/stroke/senior care. We understand the preferred resident is one who simply sits all day, looking out a window, but is that what these caregivers really signed on for? Do they really want the senior who is only a shell of a person, unable to walk, talk, or share? Did they, at least, enter into the profession with the goal of making a difference and bringing peace of mind to the elderly before they became bored with caring?

At one facility, there was a large man named Robert who never spoke. He stared at his hands, mumbled, and gave little eye contact. But one day, while talking in my sawmill-soft voice (as is my nature), Robert looked up at me and laughed at my punch line.

I lit up. "Right? Are ya with me, Robert?"

And he nodded, grinning.

I had my audience and was on a roll. "So, what's your deal?"

I began asking him questions and he answered, which was stunning to the staff.

"He never talks!"

We learned Robert stopped talking about four years prior.

But as our visits continued from one day to the next, it became clear Robert was looking for me and actively listened during our conversations.

Why?

Because he could hear me! Because I spoke directly to and engaged with him. Because I didn't just tell him what he was supposed to doing or not doing, but I interacted with him as a person. I told him jokes. I told him what was happening in the news, and I asked him about his life.

Though Robert had been in their care for years, it was I who, after just ten days, was able to tell them about Robert's career in the military, his sports background, his family, and his favorite movie. It wasn't that I possessed some great skill set. I just took the time to talk to him.

Today, I still think about Robert. Leaving him is my one regret when we moved our father again because I fear Robert has gone back to his quiet black hole where he hears nothing and he has no one to share his smiles with.

Throughout the coming months and locations, however, we were on more fact-finding missions about Daddy. *Operation What's-He-Doing-Now?* and *Operation What-Language-is-He-Speaking?* were two favorites.

One day, a very distracted caregiver appeared to be looking for something. She was polite but was also clearly worried. When I asked if everything was okay, she gave me a rather sheepish smile. She couldn't find her phone.

"And I just had it," she said, in disbelief.

We were standing, we three—with Daddy in the middle—when I suggested calling the phone and tracking the sound.

I called the number and, like a slow-motion scene from a movie, we both looked as Daddy's shirt pocket lit up and began to ring.

Keys, phones, wallets, and purses were all especially interesting to Daddy.

When I mentioned this to several former comrades of my father's, each responded in kind: *escape and evade*. It was classic military training drilled into Daddy's psyche for more than thirty-five years. It was how he was able to escape the Vietcong, the KGB, the CIA (yeah, *that* CIA), African drug lords, and guerrilla camps.

It also explained a few of the phone calls we received.

"Um, it sounds like your dad is speaking French. Does he speak French?" one nurse asked.

Yes, he does. Or he did. So, yeah, I guess he still does.

Not a week had passed before the next comment. "We're not sure but it sounds like your dad is speaking Korean or something like that."

That would be Vietnamese.

But the best was when he was still at Ennis Care and I walked in to find several nurses at the nurses' station gleefully discussing the Colonel. Their smiles brightened when they saw me and they waved me in. Apparently, he was speaking yet another language, and the nurses were trying to determine what it was. A few attempts were made to mimic him.

I smiled and repeated a few words that made them all smile in turn. Russian. As fun as it was, that was the moment one of the nurses said she believed Daddy thought he was a prisoner of war and needed to escape.

Of course!

We are, Michelle and me, the daughters of the Colonel, the White Knight, the man of many missions, and so we devised a few plans of our own. Daddy wasn't some brain-dead old man dwelling in a zombie state. He had things going on in that head of his. He was plotting, humoring people, and waiting for his big chance. And so, Michelle and I devised *Operation Door* and *Operation Pick-up* as ways to distract. We came up with *Operation Leave*, and *Operation Mom*, all of which entailed ways to manipulate Daddy into going or not going somewhere, recognizing Mom, and/or being agreeable. But *Operation Lets-Get-the-Hell-Out-Of-Here* was our favorite. Michelle, Mom, Daddy, and I were at the end of the hallway when Daddy began fiddling with the keypad at the nurses' station. We were told he had already decoded it twice before and almost escaped.

On this day, however, Mom was not having it and began pulling on his arm.

They began wrestling over it, and I was moving to intervene when they pulled the thing off the wall.

We looked at each other, then gaped at the spot formerly occupied by a security keypad.

Daddy exalted.

One of the sterner nurses was coming down the corridor, and Michelle panicked. "Let's get the hell out of here."

Now, this is a bold statement. This implies swiftness. This suggests quick movements and fast feet.

Michelle and I looked at each other then at Daddy.

Michelle whispered in Daddy's ear, "Incoming. We've got incoming!"

We each grabbed an elbow and hustled Daddy around the corner, into another resident's room, and behind the door.

And damned if Mom didn't move out like an Olympic sprinter.

We all flattened ourselves against the wall as we heard the nurse. "What the—?"

We delighted in our escape.

Michelle poked her chin at Mom approvingly. "Nice footwork, Mom."

Mom beamed.

At the new location, however, the laughs were fewer and further between. This brought on the additional stress of paying an outside company to sit with our dad and the beginning of our financial ruin as we paid approximately seventeen thousand dollars for three consecutive months while the caregivers couldn't be bothered to work for their pay.

We considered *Operation Beat-the-Shit-Out-of-These-Worthless-Women*, but…there were more problems than positives so, we just bitched a lot.

Less than forty-eight hours after burying Aunt Elizabeth, Daddy had almost finished himself off in the same manner.

I looked at Michelle, but Michelle was staring at the floor.

There was a sudden shift in our medical attention. It was subtle but it was there. He had come in a feeble old man with a serious head trauma. Now he was just a drunk.

Mom was in utter despair, crying softly and wringing her hands, uncertain what she should do.

I was pissed because he was doing this to me—to *us*—again.

What I am about to say is not fair as he has a disease, but I'm being completely honest. I was pissed because when life had gotten hard, once again, he'd tried to check out by way of blind drunkenness, family be damned.

But while I brooded and Mom shrank away, Michelle set her jaw. She'd felt the shift as well, and she was not about to tolerate anyone in that hospital writing her dad off as a drunk.

She followed the nurse into the hallway and made sure it was clear that he had a medical condition, he had a procedure coming in just four more days that would relieve all his problems, and she needed them—the medical team—to set him right so he could have that procedure done. She called doctors, followed up medication requests, and arranged for Daddy's transportation to Dallas Methodist Hospital so he would already be in the very hospital where the hydrocephalus procedure was scheduled to be performed. She was his voice. She was his knight.

In the meantime, however, he was put on Librium to safely help him through alcohol withdrawals. Only later did we discover that Librium is *not* to be given to a patient with acute narrow-angle glaucoma or a mental state where contact with reality is lost. Like, for a guy with diagnosed glaucoma? A guy who with water on the brain? A guy who with reported white spots on his brain? A guy with dementia? You mean, for a guy with anosognosia?

To be fair, by the time Daddy reached the end of his stay at this facility, he had pulled a combined number of three fire alarms, knocked out a window, hit a few people, jimmied the security keypads on two different doors, and routinely upset the Alzheimer's apple cart.

We promised we would never name specific sources, but sitters from the private company began telling Michelle and me stories about the level of care within the facility. Different women from different care companies at different times on different days all consistently shared the same concerns with us. *Your father is not getting proper care. Your father is being left to sit in his own urine and fecal matter. Your father is walking unsupervised.*

I know now that it took us far longer than it should have to say something, but at the time, we were so afraid of our parents being turned out, so afraid of having no way to care for them, and so afraid to speak out that we had become as voiceless as our parents and all the other residents who were (and are) ignored or denied proper love and care.

One week after we finally brought a complaint to the management, Daddy fell and was sent by ambulance to the hospital. He would not return again to that facility. It turned out to be a blessing in disguise.

But before that blessing came, though, there was just one more call. It was the worst. The most awful of all.

The call came in about 2 am. Another sitter had walked off the job, and neither Attila nor the other worthless ones wanted to deal with our father. "You need to come in."

I was getting dressed in the living room, but Robb was already awake and yelling.

"Why can't they just do their damned jobs?"

"I don't know!" I yelled back. I didn't. All I knew was that I had to go in again, in the middle of the night, because incredibly lazy women flocked to this place and a very broken system allowed them to behave this way and still get paid. Refusing to go in, I feared, would only bring further harm upon my father.

From 2:45 to 6:30 am, I wandered the halls with Daddy, talking about various things and periodically attempting to keep him out of trouble. "No, you can't do that."

"No, you can't touch that."

"No, you can't go in there."

We had a few standoffs. He would set his jaw and glare at me in frustration, as I clearly did not understand what it was he was trying to do.

Once he indicated that there was a pool (there was no pool) and he needed to go in. Another time, he pointed out a basketball (there was no basketball) and read signs.

I guided him, re-directed him, slowed him down, and re-routed him for a full two hours until he tired and finally sat down.

When he did, I found him a newspaper and listened while he read headlines out loud.

Since his second fall, Daddy has been saying, "Okay…oooookay….okay." The medical and nursing staff of every hospital and care facility he has been in has come to know this as Daddy's *oooookay* anthem. That okay is his tell that he is about to do something. When he sits and reads, he says, "…AND…" as his way of thinking a new thought. He doesn't always actually add anything to a conversation but it is his way of being part of the conversation.

A nurse and I were talking and Daddy blurted out, "AND!" just to remind us that he was right there with us, listening.

After about two hours of *ooookay* and another two of *AND*, I was able to slip out as the morning staff came in. Daddy was content with the paper and dozing.

I got home just in time to wake up Tommy for school and start the day, such as it was. But something was very wrong.

Before that morning, despite all that was going on with my parents and as exhausted as we were, I would have told anyone who asked that mine was the happiest family in the world. I knew Tommy was going through things, but we honestly believed—because he is the most polite and kindest kid you'll ever meet—it was teenage angst.

In the past year, Tommy had all kinds of growing pains and was constantly aching. I had him tested for everything ranging from Lyme disease to lupus and even had blood work done for possible cancer. We couldn't figure out why he was in so much pain. Beyond the body aches with no known cause, he was also sleeping during the day then not sleeping at night. He was upside down, but all the tests came back fine, and we thought it normal teenager stuff.

When he got into trouble with another student, it was so completely out of character for him that we were more stunned than mad. Again and again, we just said, "Tommy? Tommy Allred?" Other students had a history of such troubles, but not Tommy. We were shocked he participated. Clearly, it was a sign something was going on but he was also always our lovable Tom.

What I didn't know, until much later, was that when the phone had rung and I'd been summoned to take care of my father in the wee hours of the new day, Tommy was awake. Insomnia was a real issue for him, and he was sitting on the staircase, listening to the entire exchange between me and the facility and then me and Robb. He heard me say I couldn't take much more, complaining about how tired I was, and he heard his dad yelling about money.

Somehow, unbelievably, Tommy came to the decision that my life would be easier without having to deal with him, too. Sleep deprived and upset, he took some pills.

When I returned home, I found Tommy wearing his church clothes and laughed. He's got the best sense of humor, and I thought he was being goofy. I thought he had gone to bed wearing this outfit so he wouldn't have to dress in the morning. It was a very Tommy-like thing to do, so I laughed.

But he was super grumpy. Rude even. And he's never been rude. He has never been the kind of kid who talked back or was snippy, yet he was that morning.

Little did I know, he was out of his mind from the pills.

I made him breakfast.

He was surly, but he ate, and I cleaned the kitchen.

As I did, he came over and hugged me. I figured he felt bad. I thought it was because he had realized he was being a grump and was sorry for piling on.

I told him that it meant more than he knew and thanked him.

As he walked off, I thought I heard him call my name.

I will never be able to show enough gratitude for what happened next. Because he called out once more, saying *sorry*, I was able to be there for him. Nothing else matters. I got one more chance.

I got to find my Tommy.

Depression is a deceptive, vicious, lying monster that can convince a smart, good-looking, sweet, adored child that he is worthless. While depression runs deep in our family, it never once—not once—occurred to me that it could touch Tommy. I would have told you he was such a happy kid.

As of this writing, only a small number of people know this part of our story, but with Tommy's permission, we're sharing it because we want people to understand depression. You don't get over it. You can't suck it up. Real depression doesn't work like that because it is chemical. It is

an illness that nearly destroyed us. Depression, I'm learning, is a pervasive beast…like cancer. It

sneaks in. It lies. It cheats. Even now, Tommy cannot fully understand what really happened that

morning. But I have him and that's all that matters to me. Unlike cancer—and this has to be

said—once identified, you have a far greater chance of surviving it and he has. He is thriving. He

is brilliant and when I asked him (for the fifth time) about sharing this very personal story with

strangers, his response is and has always been instant: "If it will help someone, let's do it."

He is my hero.

We also opted to share his story because it also shows how much the strain of caring for those

afflicted with dementia, Alzheimer's, and brain damage affects the entire family.

It wasn't enough that our father was suddenly brain damaged and our mother's Alzheimer's was

spiraling out of control. We also had no real grasp of the situation. Because there was no legal

standing for us with the banks, with businesses, with credit cards and, briefly, with medical, we

were all trapped inside a whirling tornado of chaos and misery with no end. This book was titled

Operation Caregivers *because* caregivers were so important at this point in our crisis. Sadly, for

us, the level of care was suspect. As our story progresses, there is a happy ending regarding care

but we share our trials so that you, the reader, might be stronger, wiser, more proactive than we

were.

I digress.

But when this unexpected twist took place with Tommy, we were blindsided and then guilt

ridden. We never saw it coming.

Even worse, I thought we were all so happy, and, I missed all the cues. Because my dad thought

he was a prisoner of war and couldn't stay still, and those lazy, worthless, money-sucking memory-care people couldn't do their jobs, and I couldn't explain to my own husband why we kept paying them for nothing, and I couldn't seem to get everything together like I should, and I wasn't managing all the daughterly responsibilities, and I was so tired…of everything…all the damned time. I did not yet have legal power of attorney and could not stop my parent's money from bleeding out of their bank accounts. We were free falling every day and praying no other catastrophe hit us. And because of all those things, I almost lost my son. Suddenly, I was standing in the very same hospital I'd been in with my father, only now I was looking at my son. Not one thing in the world made sense to me.

Kerri was teaching outside Houston, and Katie was at work in College Station when they got my call. Both dropped everything, swooping in, to be there for Tommy.

Tommy was transported to Children's Hospital while we spent much of our time asking what had happened. *Why* was our word of choice.

The only answer I came up with was that I was so pissed at my father (not fair, I know) and the inept staff of his care facility that I could barely see straight. *I almost freaking lost my son because those lards couldn't walk at a snail's pace for a few hours in the middle of the night!* No, I had been stuck in the hallways of the care facility with my father who was determined there was a pool on the other side of what was actually the bedroom door of a female resident. I was watching my father as he rattled and rattled and rattled and rattled her door until I finally slid in between the door and Daddy, and I gently pushed him backward.

He was defiant and had that look. The one I later learned came just before he lashed out. I remember hoping I could somehow get through to him. While we had tried so many times and in so many ways, I remember desperately wanting to get through to his brain—to the real Marc Powe—and ask why he was doing this.

Instead of telling him *no*, like everyone else, because he was always doing something he was not

supposed to be doing, or redirecting him because he was always into something he should not be

in, I wanted to talk to him. I honestly hoped if I looked deep enough into his eyes, I could get

through to him. He and I had a special connection. We understood each other. Growing up, it

was always Michelle and Mom on one side and me and Daddy on the other. We were the same,

he and I. We had the same work ethic, the same hard push to achieve, and the same relentless

spirit. I thought I could make something, even if only for a second, click inside that befuddled

but still-amazing brain of his, and so…I did. I asked in a quiet but stern voice, "Daddy, why are

you doing this?"

I got nothing.

His stare was as blank as ever.

All the while, my beautiful boy was making the misguided decision to ease *my* ordeal by taking

himself out of the equation.

Yeah, my rage was mighty. My focus became my son, and I did not see my father for almost

three weeks.

In the weeks that followed, I remembered that blank stare over and over. At first, it stirred up

nothing but anger. I wanted to shake my dad, tell him how all his shitty decisions in life, from

overindulging our mother to overspending money to wallowing in alcohol, had led us to this state

of absolute misery. It was his fault. All his fault! I'd almost lost Tommy because my father

couldn't say no.

I called my boss and told him I wouldn't be in for an extended period of time and, through many,

many tears, explained why. As it happened, he knew from personal experience what I was going

through, and we talked about that.

In the months that followed, while talking to the suicide prevention folks at the hospital and various counselors, I learned how very prevalent suicide is, how depression is growing, and how once depression takes hold, it can actually change and imprint the brain, making grooves in the tissue. I would say that's fascinating—and, from a medical standpoint, it is—but I found it horrifying. If I or any of the army of doctors Tommy saw during the past year and a half had only seen this, maybe one of us could have headed it off somewhere along the way.

Instead, my constant whining and complaining about my parents' situation had been piling on Tommy and I was oblivious.

For a long while, we told almost no one what happened. We didn't want Tommy to be stigmatized for something that, turned out, was chemical and beyond his control. We wanted the world to view Tommy as he used to be and was meant to be—a brilliant, sweet, kind-hearted kid who is funny and charming and silly. Sharing was hard because I didn't want him to be thought of as the kid who tried to end it all.

He should be thought of as the kid who is going to *be* it all!

By the time Daddy fell again and was taken to the hospital and then another facility, I was numb. My focus remained on Tommy.

We went through counseling as a family and never had I been prouder of my girls. Therapists and counselors remarked how close we were, how fun and funny we were together, and all the things I'd *thought* we were before. There was an undeniable irony in that it took great trauma to bring us together in the exact way we'd always wanted to be.

And Michelle…

Somehow, Michelle managed to be there both for and with our mother and father.

Looking back on it now, I do not know when she slept or ate. I cannot imagine how she functioned.

We started game nights, movie nights, and refocused on the family—which was how it should have always been anyway but life and work and Robb's travel and my parents had all gotten in the way. We discovered the game *Telestrations*, a game board version of *Telephone* but with pictures. It's hilarious and, like every game we play, we were so competitive that other families within the Children's Hospital began looking at us with some measure of concern.

The nurses, however, were highly entertained as we assaulted one another.

Far and away, Michelle Powe is the single worst drawer in the world, but Robb is a very close second. In just one example, Michelle was instructed to draw something as the sand in the game's hourglass slipped away.

Given to compulsive perfectionism, a most ridiculous concept when you're the world's worst drawer and you're drawing something, she began trying to "fix" her picture.

Time!

The picture was then passed to Kerri, an excellent artist, who was given the task of guessing what the picture was.

As Robb delighted at the most horrible picture ever, Kerri furrowed her brow.

"Um. A rapist?"

Michelle gasped. "What? No! That's Sleeping Beauty!"

Tommy, Robb, and the girls fell over laughing, and Michelle joined them.

For me, it was a moment. I was watching my sister, diagnosed with chronic depression, sufferer of severe migraines, two broken necks, a battery of health issues, and a survivor of a full-blown addiction, laughing at her own horrific rendition of Sleeping Beauty. She was operating on almost no sleep but she was here. For us. For Tommy. This was family. This was what life was all about.

Reconnecting remains one of the best and finest moments of my life.

While we were healing, we were also preparing for a wedding and an audition on *Shark Tank*. Amazingly, it was Tommy who held us together.

In 2013, I began teaching fitness classes for free to a group of special needs young adults. With each class, I fell a little more in love with each of them and watched them make their way over hurdles they'd never been challenged with before. I also began to recognize different movement patterns and inefficiencies. After twenty-five years in the fitness industry, I was able to see what functional movement truly was and, for the first time, understood why it was so important as I worked with young adults with cerebral palsy, down syndrome, autism, stroke/seizure victims, and those with developmental and intellectual disabilities. Teaching steps that many others in the so-called *normal* classes might have seen as simple was fascinating, rewarding and, I realized, greatly needed. It inspired me to create an exercise program for those with special needs, which evolved into a program helping those with Parkinson's Disease and the senior population as well. Tasks like leaning over a sink to brush teeth or reaching overhead to remove something from a shelf were nearly impossible for some but, with many, could be improved or corrected.

Ironically, it included the future needs of my parents.

By the spring of 2016, I had arranged to audition my concept and product before a *Shark Tank* producer but, given all that had happened, decided against it.

Just a few weeks after, my eldest child, Kerri, was to be married. Like me, she began to ponder if elopement or a simple ceremony before the Justice of the Peace wasn't the better solution.

On both counts, Tommy insisted we carry on.

So, we did.

Shark Tank was a bust. At least, this was my initial thought. The twenty-something producer we spoke with was far more interested in products that had to do with alcohol, beauty, and fashion. While family and friends watched Jamie, one of my students, and I give our pitch, they later concurred that our producer wasn't even listening.

Special Needs ain't sexy.

Now, however, I couldn't be more grateful. Had she actually cared and had we been selected, it would have piled on a new kind of stress we simply weren't ready to incur. Today, we are the better for it.

And though it could be argued that nothing went right with Kerri's wedding, by golly, that too ended up being perfect in its own way.

Just before Kerri and Kyle's wedding, while standing in Mom's kitchen, I fielded a most unusual phone call from a young captain in the U.S. Army. As happened so often, it was up to Michelle or I to answer a phone that would have otherwise never been answered.

The voice on the other line asked to speak to Colonel Powe.

I was in the midst of fighting for legal standing in my father's legal affairs, so I was hesitant to say that my father was living in a memory-care facility. Instead, I asked who was calling and learned that Captain Kenneth King had been calling the house for many months only to be told by Mrs. Powe (Mom), the Colonel was not available.

"I am a Captain in the Military Intelligence Corps of the Army. In July, I begin Intermediate Level Education (ILE) and (around that time) will be promoted to major. However, as a part of ILE, I will be getting my master's in military history, and one of the requirements to graduate is a fifty to one-hundred-and-twenty-five-page thesis. So, after discussing this with one of the professors at ILE, I decided I wanted to write about how the military intelligence company (MICO) was formed, what decisions were made along the way, from the 50s to present day, that determined how MICO was organized the way it is."

When King began searching *integrated combat intelligence system*, he found information in a 1973 publication of "The Evolution of American Military Intelligence" about the Korean War by Marc Powe. In fact, King found numerous articles, but it was an article in *U.S. Army Intelligence History: Sourcebook*, published in 1995, titled "Which Way for Tactical Intelligence After Vietnam?" that sent King on the hunt to find our dad.

"At that point, I began to search specifically for who your father was. I found a profile on LinkedIn, and basically, from there was able to track down the phone number to your parents' house.

"I think I started calling in January every two or three weeks or so. Your mother was very nice but always regretted that your father wasn't in. I was lucky to catch you."

Indeed.

Throughout the next week, I packed box after box of files Daddy had acquired over his decades of research.

Just days before the Kerri and Kyle's nuptials, my childhood friend who had flown in for the wedding, Karin Stanton, and I mailed them off. Karin, a British national (who missed her calling as a comedian), kept half sheltering, half hiding the boxes each time a person walked near.

"Can we be doing this?" she kept whispering. She had seen the files. She saw the red CLASSIFIED stamps across several of the covers and, knowing my father since our days in Moscow, could not believe we were using a standard delivery service to send them away. "Isn't this a federal crime or something? Is this treason?"

"No! I'm sending it to an Army captain!" I had done my due diligence and communicated with the appropriate authorities to learn what could be shipped.

Still, Karin wasn't convinced we wouldn't be arrested or that this wasn't somehow an elaborate scheme by the Russians to gain access to outdated military intelligence research material.

Oh, those Russians. Almost a year later, to the day, King sent me an email from Lori Tagg, the Command Historian at Fort Huachuca where Daddy had been inducted into the Defense Intelligence Hall of Fame.

Another article from Daddy had been discovered.

"Most of the data your dad has, I haven't been able to find anywhere else."

Daddy's intel had not been filed in the Fort Huachuca Library, the Combined Arms Library, nor had it been found in the National Archives or at the War College. The boxes of paperwork we'd sent was a treasure trove of information.

"I really wish I could have talked to your dad," King said. "This is exactly what I am writing about."

While I understood King's disappointment, he had no idea how pleased we all were to be able to hand material over that allowed him to continue Daddy's work but also, I hoped, become the kind of intelligence officer that would have made our father so proud.

With much of Daddy's files sitting in the hands it needed to be in, it was time to turn our attentions back to the wedding at hand. In what was quickly becoming standard operating procedure for us, the night before Kerri's wedding was one that would have sent most people packing. For us, it was just another night.

Look at us! You can poop all over us, Fates. We don't care!

We learned the church had changed our reception area from a large gymnasium that held two hundred and fifty people easily, with open airways and a giant dance floor, to a very small room that held one hundred people, crammed, and no place to dance. Additionally, the church had decided to fix the air-conditioning units, forgetting about our wedding date, and would offer no A/C on the day of the wedding. Kerri's bridal shower was a bust with sick bridesmaids, and as if on cue, Daddy fell again. This marked his seventh significant blow to the head.

At exactly 9 pm, the evening before Kerri's big day, Katie, our middle child, ended up with a sudden dog emergency. Her giant Doberman pinscher had been gnawing on a circle-shaped soup bone when it slipped over his lower fangs and was now stuck.

We called Emergency Pet to learn that it would cost about six hundred dollars to remove the bone.

How much more were we supposed to take? Just how much hell were we to endure?

The look on Kerri's face was heartbreaking.

That was when I looked at Karin Stanton, who is also a pet sitter, and asked, "How much melatonin do you think it would take to knock him [Doberman] out?"

Children's Hospital had recommended Tommy take the natural sleeping aid for his insomnia, so with a significant number of pills on hand, we doped that Dobie up and watched him slump into a stupor as Robb and Michelle took bolt cutters to the bone and Dozier's face.

When the bone split in half and clunked to the ground, we all leapt to our feet, hands over our heads, and whooped in triumph. We high-fived and danced! No doubt, neighbors thought we were having a party what with all the cheering and carrying on.

We were. We needed that victory so badly, and thanks to the grand efforts of our new in-law family, the Beckmans made sure the wedding went off without a hitch.

Still, the day was a trial for Tommy—still struggling with some depression—and it was hard on Mom, who was disoriented and angry. Never had any of us imagined Kerri and Kyle getting married without their Papa being there to witness it.

Two days later, I woke to too many texts to count. The messages spanned everything from, "Where are you!?" and "Are you okay?" to "CALL ME!"

Panic flooded my heart, and my mind went straight to Tommy. I knew for certain he was okay, though. I had just looked at him.

Next, my thoughts went to my father. *He's fallen. He escaped. He hurt someone. Or someone hurt him.* But as I looked at text upon text sent from friends near and far, I was confused. *How would any of these people—one in Virginia, another in California—know about my father before I did?*

As it happened, a local fitness instructor had been brutally murdered in Midlothian, during the early hours of April 18th, 2016. Many knew I taught 5 am classes and was known to be up and out of the house by 4:30. Most did not know I had given up the majority of my classes and slept in that morning to be near Tommy.

I knew the instructor. Missy Bevers and I met, and she ended up a student in one of my self-defense classes before her death.

Her murder was a horrific shock, which rocked our small community, and remains unsolved, despite quite a bit of evidence. It made national news, and everyone had an opinion. There was plenty of dirty laundry aired, which resulted in far too much finger-pointing. Missy definitely made some bad decisions in her life, but she did not deserve to be vilified, especially following a very terrifying, painful, and undeserved death.

As we all learned the details, I spent more time thinking about her family than her murderer. Blaming someone for something they can no longer control or rectify does no good. There was no comfort in holding a grudge and I could not help but look inward.

I had a writing career and was starting a business for special needs. I was teaching, both for the gym and the college, and helping other authors, but my number one job was being a parent. It was the single most important thing in my life.

Robb stopped traveling and the girls were splitting time—Kerri coming home on the weekends and Katie during the week—to remind Tommy what was most important. Life.

While our Tommy of old was slowly coming back to us, we were losing Daddy, and in the midst of chaos, I found great clarity. It was time to see my dad again.

Chapter Eight

October 2016

> *Those "awful white girls" had picked up Mom at the memory care and asked how she was doing and she'd said she was good, except she really didn't care for those "awful white girls." In fact, she really didn't like one young woman she described as* snotty and rude, *and who happens to be white.*
> *Alex: Well, it's just the one, right?*
> *Mom: No! There is a whole pack of 'em.*
> *Later in Walmart...*
> *Alex: [I quickly ushered Mom to the side and pointed from the chips and nuts aisle.] Look out, Mom! There's a pack of white girls!*
> *[There were four of 'em. We eyed them suspiciously]*
> *Mom: Well, they're acting fine now...*
> *I wasn't sure if she was kidding or not...so I watched 'em extra close, just to be sure.]*

I don't recommend automatic bank withdrawals for anything. It's easy and convenient until there is an accident, until there is an emergency, until something happens that otherwise distracts loved ones from knowing what and when and how you were doing business.

In our case, despite having my father's email password and an ability to monitor much of his online correspondence, I couldn't stop the auto withdrawals from his bank accounts. National Pet Insurance, several cosmetic companies, a magazine company, two different computer software companies, and a couple more military-based organizations were all taking money each and every month, and I could do nothing.

One of the political camps was back, once again helping itself to the tune of two hundred and fifty dollars a month. A PBS station in Washington D.C. popped back up, taking their share, and yet another Native American Indian tribe decided to dip into the accounts as well.

As it turned out, I had legal standing. I was named executrix of the will. I had medical authority. Yet, I could not stop them from taking of my parents' money. *How can this still be happening?* I knew for a fact that I had spoken to many of these representatives on the phone, sent emails to some, and for a few more I had sent actual hard copies through the mail as I had to prove that I was who I said I was by showing Power of Attorney paperwork.

Two major problems were working against me from the get-go.

First, identity theft is a global issue of epic proportions, costing billions of dollars of damage in national and international businesses. Even with proper paperwork, there is very little trust. But secondly, businesses do not like losing a customer, even one who is brain damaged. At the end of the day, it isn't about Daddy's health and welfare. It is about the company's bottom line.

Companies and organizations were more than a little reluctant to work with me.

As I mentioned before, not only had Daddy set up monthly automatic withdrawals, but he also had bi-monthly, quarterly, and mid-year accounts for various fundraisers and/or billing accounts. With no paper documents to follow, we were constantly uncovering the loss of yet more money after the fact.

As the fight continued with the bank receiving our mother's social security and our father's pension checks—something we had only recently discovered—we had no idea their accounts were also slowly being drained of money by the aforementioned organizations, institutions, and companies.

What we did find out, however, was that Mom was dead.

Yeah. That was fun.

Mom and I went to Wells Fargo to ask for more assistance once we figured out money was also being taken from that account. We thought if we simply closed the account with Daddy's name on it, re-opened another account with my name on it, then I could monitor every penny.

Wells Fargo went above and beyond. They took pity on us as they watched me fumble through a thick folder of every legal document I could find naming me Power of Attorney while Mom packed and re-packed and re-packed and re-packed her purse.

Michelle and I both try so very hard not to have conversations about Mom while she is with us, as though she cannot hear or speak. We know it's demeaning. However, it is challenging as she doesn't know her own social security number, she doesn't know the date, which county we live in, or what time it is. Asking too many questions throws a red flag to the business person we are dealing with that she may not have the mental capacity to give consent for us to act on her behalf.

For a brief period, before I got legal documentation naming me her POA, I artfully danced around those questions, giving the appearance that Mom knew the answer, but in reality, I was simply answering for her. To Mom's credit, she usually nodded at the appropriate times, so we functioned well together.

But we hit a serious roadblock at Wells Fargo when they came back and told us Mom was dead…according to the Social Security Administration, at least.

Very little fazed us at this point, and I looked at Mom and said, "Wow! You look amazing." To the bank folks, I stated the obvious. "But she's not really dead."

This earned me a sweet, sympathetic look. "But Uncle Sam thinks she is."

Uncle Sam? What does he know? Still, I understood. The bank couldn't help us until we proved to the Social Security Administration, the federal government, and Uncle Sam that Mom was alive.

We went to the driver's motor bureau to renew a license because, in the throes of a 2 am Alzheimer's raid on her house, Mom had thrown it away.

Or, so we thought.

Six months after this trip, Michelle found Mom's license tucked neatly into a package of sewing needles.

Of course. Sewing needles and driver's license. Why didn't we look there from the beginning?!

Onward ho, we went to the Social Security Administration office and spent what seemed like Mom's remaining lifetime sitting in the lobby, waiting for our number to be called.

At last, it was our turn.

"What can I do for you today?"

I waved jazz hands around my mother. "This is my mother. She's not dead." I heard a chuckle somewhere behind us.

We had a discussion about how we had gotten other official identification for Mom, in spite of her apparent death, and the Social Security officer was aghast. "They recognized her, even though she's been declared dead?"

"Well, she's very lively for a corpse," I said and we all, including the guy behind us, had a good laugh.

At last, we came to the legal conclusion and documentation that my mom was, in fact, not dead. *What a relief!* "While we're here…" I was determined to get as much out of the visit as I could, "can we get my dad's social security information sent to his new address here in Texas?"

It seemed the Social Security Administration believed both parents still resided in Virginia. We established that Mom was alive and living in Texas, but it looked as if it wasn't going to be so easy for my father.

"He needs to fill out this information," the agent said.

I stared at her. I had told her no less than four times at that point Daddy was brain damaged, couldn't speak, and couldn't function without a significant amount of help, in fact.

Deep breath. "But he's brain damaged," I said, yet again.

"Can he write his name?" she asked.

"Well, yeah…"

The same woman who had just questioned another agency giving apparently the only official case of real-life *The Walking Dead* on record—my mother—documentation was suggesting I coerce my incoherent father into signing something he had no capability of understanding. "Just get him to sign this and we can turn the information over."

And that was that.

The point here is not to rat on federal government employees but to identify how random everything is and how horribly easy it is to take advantage of the elderly. There is no one rule when dealing with Power of Attorney paperwork, legal standing, or proper protocol. The entire thing is one giant crapshoot.

Many times, during the process of shutting down my father's website accounts, I was able to do so not because I faxed or scanned or mailed the proper paperwork, but because someone on the other end of the line had a parent with Alzheimer's or dementia and understood what I was going through. "Let me take care of this," became my favorite phrase in those situations. Still other times, I needed this and not that. With other exchanges, it was that and not this.

In this instance, it took me, Michelle, Mom, a caregiver, *and* a sitter helping Daddy sign the proper paperwork stating that he was of sound mind and body and needed an address change for his social security.

We got it done, but I didn't like it.

I tried to ensure that we did everything above board, but as we cajoled and bribed Daddy into signing the paperwork, I looked over at Jack, an eighty-something-year-old man who believed Jesus Christ walked with him. I don't mean figuratively, in a faith-based kind of way, but literally, in a "Hey, look who is here with me today!" kind of way, and so I said, "You see, Jack, we're doing this for all of humanity." Because who's to say Jesus Christ wasn't really there? Even though I knew it was all in the best interest for my father, it felt icky.

Seniors lose approximately $2.6 billion annually to fraud and exploitation. Over 55 percent of this financial abuse is committed by caregivers and family members. In fact, power-of-attorney abuse is the fastest rising form of financial exploitation among seniors.[1] From forgery, rerouting assets, to outright theft, it is becoming a global problem as grown children (or other relatives) unwilling to wait for an inheritance they believe is rightfully theirs, scam elderly relatives. In the United Kingdom, over 80 percent of the Crown Court cases involved fraud against elderly relatives as of 2015.[2]

Delving into the world of fighting with banks and businesses, I heard a recurring theme again and again—family members were stealing from their parents. As disgusting as it was, I was determined to make sure no one thought I was such a person.

Lest I hit my head and became deranged, I also wanted to set up a safety net for my parents so that, even if I wanted to scam them, I could not do so without alerting someone else. Hence Uncle Stephen's complete access to my parents' bank accounts. He can view them whenever he wants.

---

[1] Khalfani-Cox, Lynette, AARP, Are You a Victim of Financial Abuse? Recognize the signs – and fight back, Money Consumer Protection, March, 2011.

[2] http://www.dailymail.co.uk/news/article-3184508/Grown-children-stealing-millions-elderly-parents-frustrated-waiting-inheritance.html#ixzz4mj1Hiqb2

In this great age of technology, the value of human lives has become minimalized. What we really want to know is if our computers are working, if our social media is up-to-date, if all systems are a go, and if, and only if, the wheels of progress are turning, then we are okay. Actual individual human needs do not factor into a company's website algorithm. But get one-on-one with a person, an actual fellow human being, and the value of life increases.

In all of this, despite stories of theft and fraud, my faith in humanity remains intact.

Uncle Stephen, and even Robb, kept asking why I didn't get online to check bank statements rather than going in person to our local Wells Fargo branch. But when I go into Wells Fargo, I know everyone on sight. I don't have to tell the story of my father falling or my once-dead, now-alive mother suffering from Alzheimer's as I struggle to transfer money from one account into another to settle debts. They, my dear fellow humans, work *with* me by doing things a hardware system cannot and often will not do. We really are doing this for all of humanity.

After who knows how many hours spent on hold, waiting to discover a new password or figure out which bill was being paid by which credit card or bank, and watching the time tick away as I fought for medical records, insurance information, and legal guidance, I set up a file folder containing passwords to my various accounts—online and otherwise—and included a copy of my driver's license, social security card, birth certificate, passport, and medical information, and gathered my children together.

"This is my everything file." I made sure everyone understood, should I be placed in a memory-care facility, I do not want to be resuscitated if I stopped breathing. This was a particularly difficult—as well as personal—concept for me to share with my family, but I also laid out how I wanted my funeral handled.

Given all that we have been through, Michelle says she simply wants us to lure her out to the woods with the promise of a rare chance to see wolf puppies.

Then, she clarified—when she leans forward to peer into the freshly dug hole, she wants Robb to wallop her on the back of the head with his shovel and quickly cover her up.

In her mind's eye, this is a no harm, no foul foolproof plan when "the time comes," as she puts it, but seeing as how I'm not legally clear on what *the time comes* means (because there have been *many* times when a shovel to the back of her head seemed like a great plan), I have refused to include this in my "everything file."

Also, Robb is a little unclear as to why he's been volunteered to be the gravedigger, decoy, and shovel hitter. He suspects his role may be part of a much bigger plan that does not bode well for him.

But I digress.

While sitting in the bank of BB&T, after five months of legal headaches for yet another bank account, I asked the manager helping me finalize Mom's paperwork, "Do you have a living will for your family?"

Probably no more than thirty years old, she admitted her children had been named as beneficiaries on her bank accounts but, true to being so young, she had no actual will.

Despite the fact that many states can and will take custody of children under the age of eighteen until the courts can decide legal guardianship of a child if there is no living will, many parents do not make one. It is uncomfortable for most of us to think about.

In fact, as of this writing, Robb still has not relented to creating a living will. "We'll do it."

His is a line that I am sure is uttered by millions.

Tomorrow is another day and when talking about death, brain damage, critical condition, dementia, and/or Alzheimer's. Tomorrow seems like a much better day, indeed. Again, no one actually plans on a face-plant in their kitchen and becoming irreversibly brain damaged.

On January 11th, 2016, I knew something was very wrong with our father and his life choices were getting sketchier and sketchier, but it was still somehow all going to be okay.

By January 12th, our lives as we knew it were over, but we had no idea, until later, how bad it was actually going to get. I never would have guessed the long hours, the tears of frustration, the nonstop and completely useless telephone conversations with customer service representatives, bankers, doctors, insurance agents, vendors, and bill collectors coming my way. It certainly never occurred to me how much I would have to fight with Veteran Affairs given my father's impressive legacy with the U.S. Army. We had no idea our father had set up bank accounts in different institutions to receive different pension checks from different government bodies, thus making it difficult to gain access to anything. We had no idea about lawyers, financial advisors, and brokers in Virginia. All that valuable information was stored in Daddy's head.

And by January 12th, that information was gone, and we were at a loss.

I prided myself on being tough, yet by May, I was breaking down in front of bank and store managers, hospital directors, doctors, insurance agents, and cable TV operators. The thought of my children, any of my children, going through this was so upsetting that I began to almost obsess about all the things I needed to tell them. *Okay, if something happens to me, this is what I want you to do with....*

In my file, I listed all the friends I wanted informed of my current medical situation. I knew the list might change a little thirty years from now—ever the optimist—when my kids would actually need access to my file, but it felt better knowing I'd made my friend list. One obsession abated.

After accessing Daddy's email, I also had the unhappy task of randomly finding salutary notes from former co-workers, neighbors, and friends. My replies all began, "I am sorry to tell you this…" and I would introduce myself and explain why I had access to my father's account.

Every person on my list knows my children by name, they know my children socially, and my children know and are comfortable with my friends and co-workers. This is, I understand, more for me than my children at this point, but if I've learned nothing else, I've learned that we really don't know what our future holds. None of us do. My hope is, by including my children in all aspects of my life, there are no surprises.

During all this, Daddy ended up going to two more places before we found yet another facility we hoped to make a permanent home. Each move riled him up again, and in his confusion and agitation, the fight started all over.

With the last move, I looked at Michelle and said, "This is it. We aren't moving him again." The location was terrible (for us) but we liked the staff—genuinely. The move was hard but the room was great.

While Daddy continued his walkabouts, rattling doorknobs, and constant need to escape, he seemed to settle down. He was allowed to walk outside and sit in a closed backyard which made him happy. It made us happy too.

One day while we were all visiting, the alarm went off.

Michelle and I looked around. We knew that sound. That was the sound of Marc Powe escaping and evading. But…

He was sitting on a recliner chair between us.

We looked at him. We looked at each other. Then we looked out the back window to see the new guy, Don, trying to heft himself over the back fence by way of an overturned trashcan.

Michelle and I grinned at each other.

Oh, yeah! For once, it's not Daddy!

While nurses wrestled Don off the back fence, we high-fived. Things were looking up!

Then Mom called the police on us.

We had decided we were going to super decorate Daddy's room. This included his beloved Russian chair from our parents' house.

We rented a van and began packing stuff that meant something to Daddy and might spur a memory.

In hindsight, we should have recognized our flurry of activity and moving her things in her home would set her off. How could we not remember Mom's Alzheimer's was not okay with *flurry* and *activity* and *stuff moving*?

As Michelle and I attempted to move the Russian chair, Mom whirled.

Yeah. She whirled.

Why didn't we recognize the whirl?

Oh, wait…because we're delusional from exhaustion!

Anyway, she whirled and promptly informed us that we were *not* going to take the Russian chair. The chair was staying put.

That was it. I was tired of fighting with my parents, with everyone else on behalf of my parents, but mostly, I was just so tired.

Since March of 2016, I'd taken to walking my house in the dark of night, restless and needing assurances that all was well with everyone. My rationale was, in the event Tommy had an insomnia attack or a call came in about Daddy or from Michelle regarding Mom, I would be ready.

I was giving everything I had to everyone I loved and I was so beat down by the fact that I couldn't even give attention to my father because of my mother. I was so gosh-damned frustrated by her pack rat, hoarding Alzheimer's tendencies. *This is not about you, Karen! This is about Daddy. Sorry to say, but you can't always have everything your gosh-damned way all the gosh-damned time!* I exploded. "This is for Daddy!"

She said she was going to call the police.

Yeah. Right. I was mad. I was beyond done. I was tired of waiting on her, hand and foot. I was exhausted from driving her everywhere, back and forth, only to have her remember nothing. I was tired of her demands and wants and needs as Daddy's brain turned to mush all while I felt as if I was the one going insane as I tried to figure out where all the bank accounts were.

Ladies and gentlemen, do you want to know what you do *not* say to a person with Alzheimer's? Pay attention, because this is it. You don't say, "Go ahead. Call the police."

Don't do that.

It took Michelle and me awhile to figure out arguing and reasoning with a person with dementia is pointless. Truly. It took us more time than I like to admit to acknowledge too much activity is too much. This is a problem because if Michelle and I were to return to Earth in bird form, we would appear as hummingbirds. We've had to learn to dial our energy down, just a little, before we can reasonably help our mother (and father).

I tend to talk too loud, too fast, and meandering is a form of punishment for me, while Michelle is a compulsive straightener. She can't help herself. An unmade bed equals whirlwind activity around the entire room until it's thoroughly cleaned. A shoe on the ground requires a complete overhaul of Mom's closet.

So, Daddy needed another chair in his room?

Let's rent a truck and move half the things in his house to his new room! At warp speed! And right in front of Mom!

Yeah, sure. Nothing could possibly go wrong.

The police came and, fortunately for us, they figured out pretty quickly how confused Mom was.

It helped speed the process along when she told them we were all living in Maryland.

Still, I have managed to go my entire life without the po-po being called on me—which, if you factor in some of my activities, is pretty extraordinary—only to have my Mom rat me out.

In the end, we had to leave the Russian chair behind and vacate the premises.

The police stayed behind, watching us skulk away, while Michelle muttered under her breath that only a stupid person would challenge an angry Alzheimer's patient to call the police.

As we got into the truck, we just had to laugh about it.

Well, I think that went really well…

Ten Ways to Best Communicate with a Person Who Has Dementia

1. **Understand the disease**

    Had we taken the time to read more about what was going on with Mom, we would have understood what we were doing was frightening. Even though Mom was right there with us when the conversation of moving Daddy's Russian chair came up, she never understood. People with dementia do not process information well.

2. **No white noise**

    People with Alzheimer's and other forms of dementia cannot process information with multiple things happening. Later, you will read about us taking a virtual tour of dementia. What we learned is how confusing the entire world becomes. Remove distractions so your loved one can focus on one thing at a time. It took several outings before we figured out restaurants were terribly frustrating for Mom.

3. **Speak loud and proud**

    No one likes to be spoken to as though they are a child or poor and pathetic. Speak to your loved one just as you always have. Tell jokes, tease with love, and compliment with sincerity.

4. **Listen**

    As Mom's Alzheimer's ramped up, her voice faded. Even as Michelle and I tried to get her to speak up, Mom insisted she was yelling. The reality was she was whispering. Two things: Continue trying to make your loved one use their voice to project sound, but also really listen to what they are saying. Too many times, we simply gave up trying to hear her and stopped listening.

5. **Slow down**

    Again, this was tough for us. Keep things simple. Be still. Don't rearrange items. Just let things be as they are.

6. **Non-verbal cues**

    People suffering from dementia have a difficult time staying in the moment. They are often lost in group settings and conversations, which can make something as simple as sharing a story or giving instructions confusing and frustrating. When talking to them (or anyone else), be visual. Physical gestures (or *cuing*) help them follow along and understand what is going on.

7. **Verbal cues**

While telling a story, throw in clues to help your loved one follow along. "We went to Mary's house. Mom, you remember Mary? She lives in that big yellow house over there by the grocery store. It has the big trees in front? Yeah. That one. Anyway…" And use names. Also, stories with too many pronouns (he/she/they) becomes confusing.

8. **Don't argue or use reason**

Imagine telling a person you flew to Mars and back in one day and expecting them to believe you. For many people with dementia, your logic might as well be a story about your trip to Mars.

But what if I showed you pictures of Mars? Would you believe me then?

I don't know how many times I came home to tell Robb a story regarding Mom, and he said, "Next time take pictures and show it to her."

For us, pictures were very helpful in the beginning. For Daddy, pictures of his own personal history meant very little to him. Part of his head trauma was a social disconnect. He had very little empathy or show of emotion. Still, books about history intrigued him and pictures of helicopters and army tanks and vast landscapes caught his attention. These things brought him a sense of peace and, again, when he felt peace, we felt a little more peace.

We found picture after picture that took Mom back to a place and time that was pleasant. When she relaxed, we relaxed.

But…for the diseased brain that is under siege, photographs can be an unfair torment. She is already confused. Showing her pictures that defy what she believes to be true only increases agitation. Pick your battles. In a situation like this, let it go.

9. **Take a deep breath**

Getting anxious or uptight with your loved one because s/he can't process what is happening only makes things worse for both of you. You might have to reassess your relationship.

Growing up, Michelle and Mom always argued. It was an essential aspect of their relationship. Now, however, arguing is pointless. Coming to these terms was extremely difficult for Michelle as she lost her sparring partner.

Remember, this is not a conscious or willful action, even though it sure does feel like it sometimes! It is also a progressive disease, so it is only going to worsen. You will have to find new ways of communication that are fair for your loved one. Take a breath, remind yourself how much you love this person, and find a way to resolve whatever issues may be going on that will make him or her feel safe and more secure.

10. **Take the good with the bad**

Again, this is a progressive disease. You will have very good days and very, *very* bad ones. As time goes on, you will learn to redefine what *good* and *bad* mean. Focus on the good, understand the bad, and celebrate the life.

It was *great* seeing Don heft himself over the back fence and wrestle with caregivers instead of Daddy.

Not one month after the Russian chair/police challenge, there was another late-night call. Daddy had fallen again, and Michelle was tipped off by the EMTs that, at the time of his fall, there had only been one night-staff person on site along with several children asleep in sleeping bags spread across the floor of the facility. And this wasn't the first time.

As much as we liked her, this was not okay. Daddy was an all-hands-on-deck kind of guy. Don might be climbing over the back fence but you better believe Daddy was trying to break the security keypads and walk out the front door.

Yet, we did not lodge a complaint.

Again, when your father is essentially mute, you fear for his safety on a whole new level. Some of the caregivers were a bit on the rough side, and we worried there might be retribution taken against our father if we complained.

Instead, we convinced ourselves that she, a single mom, had probably fallen on hard times and so we tried to be understanding, despite the fact that we were paying five thousand dollars a month to now be *her* babysitter.

Anyway, we had bigger problems.

Mom was becoming increasingly dangerous in her own home, opening doors, talking to strangers, and leaving things unattended. She believed a pack of wild dogs were in the house with her when she was alone, and while we desperately tried to always have someone with her, it was sometimes impossible. A scary incident with the garbage disposal was our final wake-up call.

Mom decided (brought about by some brilliant strategy play from Michelle) she was ready to live with Daddy. It was an emotional move, more so for Michelle than me, but the timing was right. Initially, Mom and Daddy seemed happy. Daddy didn't really know who Mom was, but he seemed calmed by her. Somewhere in the fogginess of his brain, I thought he knew he knew her. The staff continuously remarked how sweet Mom and Daddy were together. They slept together, napped together, read the morning paper together.

But the move to the memory-care facility befuddled Mom's already murky memory. She was convinced there was a basement (there is no basement) in which people with guns dwelled. She was also convinced Daddy had a mistress and was leaving her. It didn't matter how many times Michelle and I told her there was no way Daddy would or could ever leave her, she would lean in and whisper conspiratorially, "You have no idea what he is like when you're not here."

Daddy couldn't string four words together, but in her mind, Daddy was filling journals with his words of love for a new young girl, his own discontent with his wife, and plans for how he was going to leave, and we could not convince Mom otherwise.

And as progressive as Alzheimer's was, bank accounts continued to be hit by unwelcomed solicitors and scammers. Any chance of Mom helping me decipher secret passwords or even answers to the security questions on Daddy's numerous accounts was gone. The push-pull, tug-of-emotional-legal-financial-we're-sorry-we-can't-help-you-war was mounting, and *Operation Bring Daddy to the Bank* was forming in our minds.

Chapter Nine

FACEBOOK: *November 2016*

Fact: You cannot reason with dementia patients (father).
Fact: You cannot reason with Alzheimer's patients (mother).
Fact: Some might think taking mother and father for a trip to Starbucks unwise...

And so it went: getting into loaded into the car, while slow going with unstable footing, was a success. We got Frappuccino's (parents fave) and pumpkin loaves, and they happily munched until our return.

Fact: You cannot reason with dementia patients.
Fact: You cannot reason with Alzheimer's patients.
Fact: The statement, "We're here!" means nothing.

And so it went: Mom was confused about the entire concept of exiting the car while Daddy refused altogether, even when I picked up his legs and tried to maneuver him. He took off his shoes.
Alex: No. Wait. Daddy, don't. Mom, where are you going? [I gathered the cuffs of my
           dad's pant legs in one hand and swung him forward.]
Mom: Where are the car keys?
Alex: [Contains hysterical laughter at prospect of Mom driving while continuing to
           wrestle Daddy] Can you go get help from the caregivers? [Whom I can see
           staring out the window at us.]
Mom walks off, forgets what she was supposed to ask.
Alex: [Gets Dad out of car but he's headed for driver's seat. I lock car door but my auto
           keycard helpfully unlocks the car for him.
He gets in.
I get him out. I lock door.
Car helpfully unlocks again.
Mom is standing by the flowerbed looking at trees.
Dad makes move for car again.
I lunge. Lock!
Unlock!
Lock!
Unlock!
Alex: Sonofa....[I throw car keys far away from me, Dad, and car.]
They land in flowerbed.
Mom: Oh, keys!
Alex: Mom...no!

On July 15th, 2016, I completely lost it. I'm talking over the edge, 'round the bend, hard core lost it.

I try to handle my parents' affairs when my kids are not around so they don't hear my rants as I fight with yet another agency, another business…another mindless corporation. Every day is like walking on eggshells, half-expecting a call about Daddy falling or hitting someone or getting a call about Mom being pushed by Daddy or having a meltdown. Even the best of days could be just one phone call away from ruin. I keep things in check by using Michelle and Robb as my sounding boards for advice, but July 15th was a day that had been building for some time. That day I hit my *done* point.

I had received notification from BB&T Bank granting access, at long last, to Mom's account. Before I could even access that account, however, I got another notification the check I had written for our parents' care facility had bounced.

Back in January, I had lost my assistance gathering information about Mom and Daddy's previous health care bills when Michelle had plummeted into a deep depression after taking on the task of going through all of Mom and Daddy's paperwork at the house. Mom never threw a single piece of paper away and so there had been decades of letters, bills, resumes, piles and piles of to-do lists, contributions, military and insurance information, magazines and newspaper clippings, and pictures.

Discovering our mother's unfulfilled dreams written out in Mom's own handwriting crushed my sister. Worse, Michelle unearthed bills spent on her during her decade of drug-induced blackout. Her guilt was all consuming. Furthermore, as new bills continued appearing at my parents' house, Michelle simply allowed the notifications to pile up without mentioning anything to me. I knew we had fallen behind in paperwork for the VA, but I wasn't aware of some important bank notices awaiting attention.

Somewhere during that time, my uncle got a peek into the account while he was with our mom. He believed there was enough money to cover at least few more months of care while we waited for New York Life to begin paying for long-term care, and I thought we finally had things under financial control. Sure, New York Life needed proof of the days Daddy had spent in different care facilities to apply them toward the one-hundred-and-eighty-day requirement on his long-term contract, but while I scrounged for information, I believed we had enough cushion in the bank to cover us.

The responsibility of being Power of Attorney became too much for this Peter Pan.

I sold Mom's minivan, but just the act of turning over the title was such a hassle. I had to find the medical POA for Mom verifying Mom's personal POA to me which, in turn, verified Daddy's POA to Mom. *Around and around and around we go.* Why the standard POA from a lawyer in Virginia was good for one bank, but not another, good for one credit card, but not the car title office, began tearing me down. I was on edge all the time, ready to challenge whomever about whatever. How much longer was this going to go on?

So, when I saw the BB&T check had bounced, I held out a sliver of hope that it was just another clerk double-checking and questioning the legitimacy issue. It honestly didn't occur to me that it had finally happened—we were out of money.

BB&T cleared me, and I got online and began studying the numbers. Six months ago, we'd had over twenty thousand dollars in Mom's account, but I discovered American Express had withdrawn so much in such a short about of time that we now had a balance of just under two thousand dollars left. Of course, I couldn't access the American Express account because they didn't recognize any one of the three POAs I had. Had I been given access to the BB&T account earlier, I might have been able to head this off. Now it was too late. The money was gone.

I sat down and wrote a pleading, pathetic, have-mercy-on-us letter to New York Life, and as I typed, I just began sobbing. Enough was way, way, way beyond enough. *I don't want to be the Power of Attorney. I don't want to spend every single day playing detective with different banks or, hunting down those taking money from my parents. I don't want to be responsible for closing accounts, following up confirmations, checking savings accounts and automatic withdrawals. I don't want to be in charge of selling their cars, storing antiques, and selling off furniture to pay an electric bill.*

Initially, Michelle and I were a great team but no longer. The demon that was depression took her out of the game and suddenly, on top of my parents' legal and medical woes, I was fighting Michelle about *her* finances, *her* car insurance, and holding up her end of the deal to clean out Mom and Daddy's house. I was always on someone about something and I hated it. Simply put, the mess our father left behind was just too much.

And however hard it was on us, it was taking its toll on others as well. Daddy's brother, Uncle Stephen, arguably one of the nicest guys you'd ever meet, blew up at Aunt Diana and an old family friend over the subject of our parents' affairs in such an uncharacteristic manner that I felt the need to apologize after he stormed off.

"He didn't mean that." I knew he didn't.

While Mom was an only child, Daddy was the oldest of five children. His siblings, known to all as hilarious story-tellers with re-enactments that involve great animation and drama, are equally loyal and loving. Even as Uncle Stephen set his retirement date, he etched out a schedule that would allow him to act as Daddy's financial advisor while Aunt Diana, a retired police detective, became our official information gatherer on quite literally anything and everything.

Little did I know at the time that they could not have come soon enough.

Everything—every little thing—was so convoluted and upside down that we were all beyond frustrated.

But the Veterans Affairs Office still had to enter the fray.

Uncle Stephen, as well as Aunt Diana and Uncle Chris, had been taking Daddy to the VA and attempting to "crack the code" on his different accounts, but we had reached critical mass. Getting Daddy situated in the VA system was crucial. In addition to more than ten thousand dollars' worth of memory-care fees, the pharmacy bills were as high as two thousand per month without Daddy's VA benefits.

Aunt Diana began extensive research on the subjects of Agent Orange and different chemicals our father had been exposed to while serving in Vietnam. She also checked into possible exposure in other countries throughout Africa and the Middle East in hopes of having the VA assist us. Suffice to say, this was a man who deserved to be taken care of by his country.

As Uncle Stephen stepped in to take up with fight with the VA, keeping Daddy in their system, and my parents' finances, and I'm sure his frustrations were mounting with Michelle and me. Of course, he never said one word but I could not help but feel as though Michelle and I were screwing everything up. I was not *not* divulging information to Uncle Stephen. I thought I was sparing him from further misery.

For everyone else, the task at hand was taking care of Marc and Karen. That was the whole picture. But for us, the whole picture included the four of us—the nucleus.

Marc and Karen Powe made their youngest daughter their Power of Attorney because Michelle's

legal status was a wreck. In fact, Michelle's personal finances were a wreck, and until recently,

her personal life was a wreck. Following a lifetime of undiagnosed medical issues, massive

headaches, Michelle's addiction to pain killers (a result of over-prescribing and, in my opinion,

malpractice by three different doctors), she lost everything. But, no matter how angry I was with

my parents for their mishandling of Michelle and her legal and medical woes, however frustrated

I was by their horrible financial decisions regarding Michelle, their intentions were always good.

As outsiders weighed in on what to do with Mom and Daddy's current living condition, someone

would invariably say, "You should probably sell their house."

Yeah, well, there's a problem.

When Mom was still living at home, still opening the front door and allowing anyone in, getting

lost, forgetting how to answer the phone or turn off the stove, Michelle packed up her

belongings, her four dogs, and moved out of her home of eight years to take care of Mom. There

was no place on Earth (certainly not in the immediate area) that would allow a renter with four

dogs.

Once Michelle left her house, I knew she had to stay in Mom and Daddy's house. She had no

money, no nest egg, and no credit. What she did have, however, was outstanding debt due to her

medical issues almost two decades prior.

With Mom in memory care with Daddy, it worked out well. Michelle was there to take care of

Mom's only remaining concerns—Colby and the house.

I recall once confronting Mom about delivering Michelle some tough love during the height of

Michelle's addiction, and Mom's response was that there was no way she could let Michelle hit rock bottom (the solution prescribed by most addiction counselors). She refused to allow Michelle to be without a nice home and/or the things she needed.

Selling the house meant making Michelle homeless, and I knew that that was something Marc and Karen Powe would not stand for. In fact, for all my feelings of ineptness, I knew my parents would consider that my greatest failing.

As Power of Attorney, I was obliged to act in a manner that would satisfy my parents.

In 1985, I was working outside Washington D.C., at the Erikson Modeling Agency, when a call came in. It was a Captain Somebody informing me that our dad had been taken hostage by the Kuwaiti government and I was to go to the whatever wing of the Pentagon and would be escorted to the whatever door by a Captain Someone Else to the briefing. By this time in our lives, we knew our father gathered military intelligence for the United States Army, had a brilliant career, and was highly respected for what he did and how he did it. Still, one can never be fully prepared for such a phone call and I was stunned.

To date, I truly only remember three things about that day. The first is the call itself, the second is the realization that then-President Regan would have to negotiate our father's return home in one piece, but the third is another phone call I received before leaving the agency.

Numb, I gathered my belongings and was headed out the door just as a buddy called about going clubbing. We were young and dumb and twenty-two years old, but my world had just been rocked.

I told her my dad was taken hostage by the Kuwaiti government.

There was a slight pause and then she asked, "So, we're not going out?"

Yup. That's what she said.

I never really spoke to her again. Not due to ill will so much as realizing I had nothing in

common with this person. That she could not understand the gravity of the situation was beyond

me. That perhaps my father's life was more important than our social one didn't even occur to

her, and I knew I no longer had time for her.

The day was a blur as we were given only partial details. Most of what occurred was deemed

classified and we, his family, would be told almost nothing. What we could do, however, was

just sit and wait for his return. I remembered feeling like we all needed to huddle up, be close,

take care of one another.

That's how it's always been.

But things had also changed over the years. I had my own family, with my own husband and

children. I was no longer just a daughter but a wife and mother.

As the child of a military intelligence officer, we moved frequently. By the time I was eighteen, I

had lived in more than a dozen places throughout the world. We were isolated from extended

family and only truly understood *family* as the four of us—Marc, Karen, Michelle, and Alex.

Michelle and I only got to know our aunts and uncles when we were older, and relations with

cousins, especially as kids, were difficult since most are so much younger than us.

It wasn't until our Uncle Stephen directly said, "He's my brother," that I realized how important

it was for my father's siblings to also be involved. While I was busily trying to protect my

children from the harshness of my parents' situation, I was also pushing away our extended

family members. They just lost their sister and now, in many ways, their brother as well. They

wanted to help. It was, as they all pointed out, exactly what Daddy would have done for them.

After my meltdown, I realized I was losing an essential part of me. Typically, a very happy

person by nature, I was becoming a grouch. Accepting help seemed like a pretty good idea.

I refocused on what I love—helping other people. Not only did I start spending more quality time with my parents but I also returned to the gym.

For three years prior to Daddy's fall, I had given free fitness classes to special needs young adults and had come to understand how woefully neglected this amazing population was by the very industry I loved so much—the fitness industry. The harsh reality was/is that most instructors and trainers were too intimidated to work with those with disabilities. Multiple myths surrounding those with special needs clouded both judgment and education and guess who lost out in the end?

But with all that had been going on with Mom and Daddy, there had simply been no time.

As Uncle Stephen and Aunt Diana stepped in, and thanks to the urging of many spectacular people, I began teaching again, and I found caring for others was what I was truly meant to do. Suddenly, I was re-energized and happy again. I had to find a way to bring those feelings of happiness back around to my parents.

Instead of being with my parents out of love and concern, out of joy and happiness, I had been visiting them out of a sense of obligation, total dread, and certain resentment.

Man, I have to change that.

So, in July of 2016, when Daddy fell yet again and his eye was protruding slightly from its socket, taking him to an eye exam didn't seem so daunting. We weren't going to wait around for the care facility doctor to look at it but we had to have a plan.

Communication with Daddy isn't always the greatest. To be clear, our communication is great. We're loud, use lots of hand gestures, and are clear in our directives. Daddy, on the other hand, has his own agenda. Sometimes he listens to you, most times not. Sometimes he'll take directives, most times not.

Launch *Operation Hummingbird.*

Before our latest operation could go into effect, we had to assess the situation. Daddy reading the eye chart was unlikely. Daddy sitting still in the examination room, much less taking directives from the doctor, was even more unlikely. But the more immediate and pressing issues were Daddy in public and Daddy with transportation.

Michelle bravely agreed to pick up both Mom and Daddy—alone—while I came from another direction and met them at the optometrist's office.

Happily, the trip to the office went well, and Daddy was able to read the eye chart. We still don't know if he went with the flow because the eye chart examinations were imprinted on his brain and he was on autopilot or he was interested (and that's key with Marc Powe). Also, because Dr. Reagan was former military, we wondered if that triggered a response from our father. It didn't matter. He followed the instructions.

It wasn't until we reached the lobby that things went sideways.

Daddy got that look.

Damn.

Mom whirled.

Crap.

Daddy's jaw was set. He was looking off into the distance and gently pushing us all ahead of him as though to say, "You go ahead, I'll be fine." Translation: *Get lost.*

Answer: *Operation Hummingbird.*

The key was doing something, *anything*, to distract him while, at the same time, letting him believe his movements were his idea. Michelle swarmed left, and I swarmed right.

My sister has a quiet voice. I do not.

So, as she flitted around him like a little hummingbird, ducking and weaving, circling him and gently pushing him in the proper direction, my voice was the added distraction.

We made it to the parking lot and went into full-on mode before Mom, as always, became our adversary.

She tries to "help" and inadvertently ends up in the way. Hence the reason *Operation Hummingbird* is *Operation Hummingbird* and not *Operation Rhinoceros*. We have to make sure Mom doesn't get bumped or pushed or knocked back.

Weave in. Weave out! Lots of hand gestures. Jazz hands help. Jazz hands! Jazz hands!

Michelle: Hey, no, Daddy, you need to...

Alex: HEEEY, DADDY, DO YOU WANT TO GET A DR. PEPPER?

Daddy: (slightly distracted) Hmm?

Bob and weave. Bob and weave. Gently direct Mom toward car.

Alex: (to Michelle): Quick, shut that door. He's making a move for the driver's seat.

Michelle: Daddy, do you want…

Daddy set his jaw and made his move (at quintessential turtle-like speed) toward the driver's seat.

A woman stopped in the doorway of the doctor's office to watch as Michelle and I played "Who's on first? What's on second?"

I made eye contact with Michelle. Mom is off course. I repeat…Mom is off course. The Whirler is AWOL.

Michelle swooped, re-directing Mom toward the right door.

Side note: During the last two months, we have watched, with a mixture of bemusement and sadness, Mom become more and more confused by which car door to use. Even if we walk her to the passenger side of the car, she follows us back to the driver's side. Unless we actively put her in her the passenger seat then securely close the door, there are no guarantees where she might end up. Mom has even attempted to slip inside the driver's door of the car parked next to us.

Back to Operation Hummingbird…

Alex: OR DO YOU WANT A STARBUCKS? ICE CREAM? FRAPPACHINO? OOOOO! HOW ABOUT A COFFEE? YOU LOVE COFFEE!

Mom settled in place.

Alex: Mom in place. I repeat, Mom in place!

Michelle flew back toward Daddy by way of the front of the car while I stood behind him at the passenger door on the driver's side. The trick was never actually touching him while turning him around. It all had to be his idea.

Alex: I'M THINKING ICE CREAM! (I looked at Mom sitting so pretty in the car, and if at all possible, I yelled even louder.). WHAT DO YA THINK, MOMMA? ICE CREAM?

Mom: (smiled and nodded) Oh, yes, that sounds good.

I thought about how much I love her sometimes. But Daddy couldn't hear her because she has the audibility of an asthmatic mouse, but I appreciated the effort.

Michelle: Hey, Daddy, let's…

Alex: THEN LET'S DO THIS THING! YEAH! ICE CREAM. (To Michelle, I mouthed GO!)

One should never underestimate the speed of a turtle, however, and Daddy made another determined move. It was bold. Like the Ninja Turtle he is, he made for the driver's door. Yeah, he thought he was going to drive.

Since this began, his one constant is that he is going to get into his car and drive home.

The woman at the front door pursed her lips, still watching in what we believed was morbid fascination.

Alex: SO, WHAT'S IT GOING TO BE? ICE CREAM? IT'S PRETTY DANGED HOT OUT HERE...

I was so loud that the Colonel finally turned and looked at me. I was sure he was thinking, "Please, shut up."

But in that spilt second of distraction, Michelle slid into the driver's seat and backed the car out, positioning it just so with the passenger door in our dad's direct path. Michelle, master behind the wheel, aimed it perfectly. This is when it really helps having "former bobsled pilot" on your résumé.

Alex: YOUR CHARIOT AWAITS! HERE WE GO! ICE CREAM FOR EVERYONE!!!

Daddy: Hmm. Ice cream.

We got him inside, buckled the seat belt, and I locked the door.

As Michelle roared away (Godspeed, Michelle), the woman from the doorway said, "Bless you, child. I hope no one ever has to do that for me."

I was conflicted. I was quite sure the woman meant to say she was sorry we had to work that hard just to get our father into a car. She hoped, I was fairly certain, that she never got to the point where her non-compliance was so hard on others.

I understood that. I've felt that same way on occasion.

While Michelle displayed great patience and care-giving skills, I had to work through my anger, disappointment, and frustrations with two people who, at the end of the day, were only human. The underlining of the statement is what we all think, isn't it? *I hope never to be like that because I sure as hell wouldn't want to have to take care of that.*

I have spent far too much time being mad that Michelle and I were placed in this position to begin with, but as stated previously, no one ever plans a face-plant on their kitchen floor any more than a body plans on water on the brain, dementia, and/or Alzheimer's. My parents are good people, albeit complicated and sometimes difficult, but they are good. Daddy's job dragged us to hell and back but it was also amazing, educational, life changing and rewarding. We were introduced to so many things because of our parents' curious and loving natures. They have been a positive force in this world and tried so hard to help others. Now it's our turn.

Operation Hummingbird was a success, not only because we got Daddy into the car but because it was also kind of fun. I was having fun taking care of my parents for the first time.

With the help of extended family members, Michelle and I found renewed faith, hope, and happiness. We started believing again. Things were going to be okay.

A few days later, while visiting Mom and Daddy, I was re-enacting a story which required lots of arm waving and flailing and yelling. *Jazz hands! Jazz hands!*

The caregivers and residents were all staring at me, open-mouthed, and smiling. For the caregivers, I was new entertainment. For the residents, I was someone they could actually hear. It is rumored—by my husband—I learned to whisper in a sawmill, which, however untrue, comes in super handy among the retirement sect. I see a long-term gig appearing at different retirement centers around the nation in my future. This is a great crowd.

As I stood there yelling and waving and noting, to my delight, Daddy's grin (be still my heart!), it hit me. Despite Marc and Karen Powe's imperfect behavior when we were kids, there were still those life lessons they imparted to Michelle and to me. They taught us about equality and empathy and charity. They taught us again and again about how to treat others and that life was so much more than getting. Giving, we ultimately learned, was the key to true happiness.

Dang.

Maybe they didn't suck as parents after all.

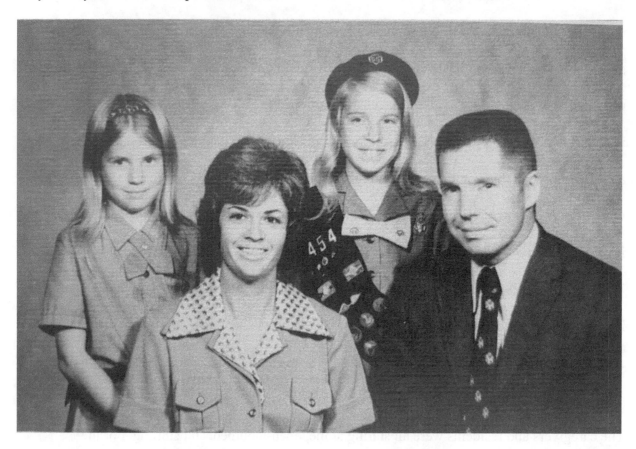

After each military family stationed in Fort Huachuca was told to have a family photo taken, this is one of the few photographs of Marc, Karen, Michelle, and Alexandra ever taken in a professional setting

Chapter Ten

FACEBOOK *December 2016*

> *Well, we finally got the safe open. It wasn't easy but it was well worth...*
> *What the what? There's nothing inside this safe but directions on how to open the safe!*
> *Are you serious?!?*

Ms. Pat had died.

I called Thurber House in Columbus to update Ms. Pat on Mom's status only to be told that she died two days prior.

It was really no shock when our Aunt Elizabeth died, and so it should have been no shock when we heard about Ms. Pat. After all, we're talking about a woman who was ninety-four years old. A two-time cancer survivor, with back, hip, and foot issues that slowed her, but she still drove, regularly attended church, participated in book clubs, socialized with the best butterflies around, and was easily the *loudest* woman in the room well into her nineties. What slowed and then ultimately stopped her was the return of cancer. I just wished cancer could know if Ms. Pat had been a spry seventy years old when it (cancer) reappeared, she would have kicked its ass all over again. Ms. Pat was *that* awesome.

So, maybe we weren't surprised as much as we were sad. Very sad.

Then came the next thought: Do we tell Mom?

Part of Mom's repetitive self-soothing behavior was saying, with a sigh, "Oh, and I really need to call Ms. Pat." Mom no longer remembered how to use a phone, certainly not alone, but the idea of talking to Ms. Pat comforted her.

But when I would suggest calling her, Mom always shrugged me off.

"Well, not right now. I can't talk to her right now."

Mom's present reality was frightening for her, so going back in time, remembering her friendship with Ms. Pat as it was, was a much safer place.

To make up for the absence of Mom's conversations with Ms. Pat, I had stayed in contact with her dear friend, but in such a short period of time, she was gone. Ms. Pat was, truly, our role model.

How to tell Mom? We moved into *Operation Ms. Pat*.

As described in several sections of this book, Ms. Pat moved herself into a retirement home. What was not discussed was how uber-aggressive she was about her retirement plans. She chose her final residence when she was fit as a fiddle and strong as an ox. She chose to take her nephew, Scott, whom she had named as Power of Attorney to her living will, to every bank, creditor, neighbor, manager of the retirement facility, and friend she could think of. She made sure everyone knew Scott's name and face so when the time came, he would have no trouble accessing vital information.

Scott later told us how uncomfortable he had been with her "when I'm no longer here, this is who you will be dealing with" plan.

But Ms. Pat wasn't going to hear it. She probably yelled at him!

I remember, about ten years ago, she called me in late October to announce she didn't want any Christmas presents. She yelled at me over the phone, which in Ms. Pat world, was merely talking sternly. "I DO NOT NEED ANYTHING ELSE! I HAVE EVERYTHING I NEED!"

Okay, a) how long had she known me? Like I was even thinking about Christmas in October, and b) the fact that she had already compiled her list of who to call and threaten was amazing, if not terrifying. But, as I sputtered and mumbled it would probably only be something like a book, as I knew how much she loved to read, she roared.

"I MEAN IT! DO NOT GET ME ANYTHING!"

I got her a book.

Still, that memory reminded me of the time she had an estate sale.

Once she made up her mind she was going to move into a retirement facility, she launched into action, hired a real estate agent and an appraiser, and had the estate sale right off.

She did it that way for two reasons. First, she wanted to ensure that all the proper people in her life had a Ms. Pat something-or-other to remember her by, and second, she wanted to raise a little money for her own retirement plan. It was a brilliant strategy as anyone and everyone who knew Ms. Pat wanted a Ms. Pat memento.

I bought, still have, and cherish an old parlor chair. I also have a few of her paintings as does Michelle, and Michelle also got a really cool library table. We all happily paid for these items knowing it was helping our dear friend.

She also did it to downsize and rid herself of things she no longer needed as she was moving from a three-bedroom house to a one-bedroom apartment. She made sure her end days would be uncluttered, uncomplicated, and worry-free.

After her husband, Charles, died, Ms. Pat reckoned she didn't want any of her loved ones to be forced to go through the emotional and/or legal stresses that she had so she devised a plan. She never called it this but hers was the original *Operation Ms. Pat.*

Today, I look back on all the things Ms. Pat did right and wished we had all taken better notes.

❖ She created a living will.

❖ She appointed a Power of Attorney, but instead of simply allowing Scott to say yes to the position, she required he meet all the creditors, vendors, and managers of her legal and financial affairs so there was always a face to the name and proper documentation of previous meetings with Scott *and* Ms. Pat. She also had him meet her doctors.

❖ She purged—every tax receipt, bill, old letter, holiday, and well-wishes card she had acquired over a lifetime. She simply let them go.

❖ She decided on her own future. After months of interviews and visits, Ms. Pat selected the home where she wanted to spend the final days of her life, prepared the proper paperwork, and awaited the proper time—precisely when *she* chose. Unlike Mom, Ms. Pat had total say in her own life, from her present to her future.

❖ She sold her home.

❖ She had an estate sale and sold all the furniture, decorations, kitchenware, pictures, unneeded or unwanted clothing and memoirs but first arranged a pre-sale with friends and family.

❖ She hired an agent to manage all the monies and debts so that she never actually took money from a friend or relative.

❖ Then, she had a kick-ass life as Queen of Thurber House, Master of the Voice, Commander of every room she was in, Life of the Party, and all-around Patricia the Great.

Ms. Pat is my idol.

With *Operation Ms. Pat* in mind, I knew it was time to have a garage sale.

Not nearly as savvy or energetic as Ms. Pat, we opted for a good old-fashioned garage sale, and my daughter, Kerri, and beautiful new son-in-law, Kyle, came into town to help.

After my children, Michelle, and I laid claim to the things we wanted, and we offered a variety of things to extended family members, we began pulling out furniture, kitchenware, pictures and frames, knickknacks, and really cool things from all around the globe. The task was much harder than expected. The act of carrying things to the lawn and driveway was simple enough. It was the letting go where we hit our snag.

The people who came to the garage sale didn't care one bit about the fact that the piece came from the Middle East or a statue was one Daddy got from the market in Mombasa, Kenya, or the vase was from the Souk, in Tunisia.

What upset Kerri most was how low I was letting things go for.

Throughout the day, I kept saying, "This is about purging, not dragging all this back into the house. We already took what was most important to us. We have to let this go."

Michelle really fought me on some of the more exotic items and things she thought meant the most to Mom. She was really struggling.

I pointed. "Look, Michelle…it is time to let go of all this."

She let go, but frequently walked back into the house and hid.

Still, as wildly successful as the garage sale was, it was an emotional ordeal.

There were so many things set outside that more than a dozen people asked if we were moving or something.

We smiled and told the story of our parents. We did so not for sympathy-sales but as a way of letting go. It was therapeutic, and the response was both beautiful and unexpected as people gave a little more cash, *always* gave a hug, and said, "I'll pray for you."

DARN THESE STUPID BUGS THAT KEEP GETTING IN MY EYES!

I was reminded of a time when Mom and I were coming back from the hospital. It was in early February, back in the days when the hopes Daddy would somehow return to us had begun to fade.

As we drove home, Mom began to softly cry and I asked what was wrong.

Asking a person who has seemingly lost everything *what's wrong?* seems so ridiculous, but I had to know.

"I wish I believed in God so I could pray."

It was a stunning statement.

Michelle and I grew up in an agnostic home. We never attended church. There were no pictures of Jesus Christ in our home, and no blessings of the food, or giving thanks to a higher power. We saluted the flag and pledged allegiance, but we didn't pray.

In the past decade, I had found faith and really liked the teachings of Jesus Christ (as documented in the book, *Swingman: What a Difference a Decade Makes*), but I had never talked about that with Mom.

I knew the power of prayer was mighty. "You could, Mom."

But she shook her head and kept crying. For her, it felt too late. It was all too late.

"Or, other people could!" I focused on the road ahead. "Lots of people already are." I couldn't explain why, but I felt it was important she knew that. "A lot of people have been praying for both you and Daddy."

It was true.

We had Muslim, Christian, and Jewish friends all praying for us. We had agnostics and atheists, in their own way, praying for us. Members of my gym family, both faculty and students, routinely asked about Mom and Daddy, always telling me they were praying for us, and on more than one occasion Michelle and I sardonically told a nurse or doctor or agent or manager to "pray for us." We needed all the help we could get.

Time and again, we were reminded of how many truly good people were out there in the world. Trust me, we needed those reminders as we watched how many others were willing to steal from and mistreat seniors.

Following the garage sale, a friend sent me a text. She had purchased a puzzle at the sale. In addition to the puzzle, my friend had also bought an antique framed mirror and a bowl. Judy had sworn the bowl held far greater monetary value than what I was asking, and I had explained it meant more to me that she loved it. It had been late in the day, and we—the children and grandchildren of Marc and Karen—had watched hundreds of people look through our parents' things as simply *stuff*. Judy Scarlett had truly appreciated the picture frame and bowl. That had meant more to us than any dollar amount she paid.

When Judy got home and opened the puzzle, she was under the ridiculous assumption that she might actually have a puzzle to put together waiting inside.

Crazy, right? It was a Marc and Karen Powe puzzle box, after all.

Michelle had checked every bag, purse, pocket, decorative box, and drawer, but it had not occurred to her to look inside a puzzle box. If she had, she wouldn't have found multiple pieces of the promised picture on the box but Mom's social security card, a Virginia driver's license, various credit cards, and even an old driver's license of our grandmother's along with various business cards and medical information.

Still, a day later came another text. Behind the antique mirror was an old picture of someone. A relative, maybe?

We are so blessed that of all the people who came by to take away our parents' things, it was this precious soul who discovered the puzzle box that wasn't really a puzzle box and what treasures the old frame really held.

One of the better surprises came not long after learning our dear Ms. Pat had died.

This was also after discovering Mom and Daddy's accounts were far lower than anyone had previously believed, and I had decided the only way we could keep Mom and Daddy safe and secure was to contact their former financial advisors out of Virginia to see if there were any stocks to sell. We needed money and we needed it fast.

By this time, New York Life was finally paying for our father, but Mom was still her waiting for own one-hundred-and-eighty-day mark.

While I was in full-blown panic mode about next month's care facility charges, Ms. Pat's nephew, Scott, called and found Michelle.

Ms. Pat had left Mom some money.

"Not a lot," Scott said, but it would hold us until October when the long-term care kicked in on their insurance policy.

What Scott called "not a lot" felt like a lifeline to us.

I could breathe again. *Thank you, Ms. Pat!*

So unexpected. So sweet. So miraculous. So Ms. Pat.

The decision to tell Mom everything came about when Mom, once again, sighed and said she really needed to talk to Ms. Pat.

I took a deep breath.

A student of mine at the gym had once told me about she and her sister reminding their mother, who had Alzheimer's and repeatedly asked where her husband was, that their father had died.

Thinking she was being helpful, my student would reply, "Mom, don't you remember? Dad died?"

Her mother would collapse into tears and sob until both sisters realized it was even more cruel to remind than not. Eventually, they simply pretended their father was tied up in traffic.

It sounded like a good plan for Mom with Ms. Pat, but Uncle Stephen reasoned this way: Even if we told her just once, we did our duty. We were truthful with our mother. Then, if/when we're all in heaven, and Mom and Ms. Pat came strolling (or floating—I'm not sure how all that's supposed to work) over to us, it would be a joyous reunion rather than, "Hey! Why didn't you tell me?"

I bet, even in Heaven, Mom will be a whirler. She'll be standing by another cloud, hear me coming, and whirl.

So, I took that deep breath and said, "Mom, there's something I have to tell you about Ms. Pat." Before I could say another word, Mom began to cry. She knew.

And she cried again when I presented Mom with the check from Ms. Pat's estate. She cried because she was so grateful, so humbled, and she so missed her dearest friend.

Mom can't hold a thought from one minute to the next, but she has consistently remembered that sweet Ms. Pat is no longer here. The mind is such a funny and complicated thing. Which is yet another reason why there is no predicting how Mom's moods are going to be from one day to the next.

By mid-summer, we had moved Mom and Daddy again. A second incident had occurred, in which Daddy had fallen, the ambulance had come out and, again, reported back that children were sleeping on the floor of the care facility.

We called the manager, but rather than leaving that company altogether, we relocated to another facility under the same owner. Once again, our hopes were high.

Mom's results were immediate. Some days she burst into tears, sure that something horrible had happened to us and she was never going to see us again. Other times, more often than not, she was just angry.

The greetings typically went along these lines:

Alex: Hi, Momma! You look cute.

Mom: Yeah. Well. Let me tell you what's going on…

She would launch into the same storyline with Michelle and me, but with different twists and turns. The staff didn't like her. The staff was mad at her. The staff was mean to Daddy. Daddy was leaving her. Daddy had a girlfriend and was going to divorce her. She went down to the basement to talk to the administrators, but they wouldn't talk to her. There were no basements but she was determined they existed. Or, sometimes, they had guns. We have never been gun owners, yet Mom was suddenly obsessed with guns.

One day I decided to try a new tactic. I took Mom by her shoulders and looked deeply into her eyes. "I didn't want to tell you this. In fact, I've been trying very hard not to tell you this." I drew in a long breath, and she truly looked worried. "Daddy is crazy. He's off his rocker. He's nuts. Really, he's nuts. So, when he tells you he's leaving you and has a girlfriend and all that, he has no idea what he's talking about."

She was used to everyone denying Daddy would ever leave her based on the sheer fact that he couldn't even talk. In her mind, she had full-blown conversations with Daddy, yet no one believed her. Suddenly, I was. For the first time, she considered it. "So, that's why Michelle and I set up a bank account that is yours and yours only. Mom, you have all the money. All the money is in your name so there is no way he could leave you."

That really caught her attention.

I piled on. "He has no car, no phone, no Internet connection. You control everything. At least, everything is in your name, and I'm kind of behind the scenes controlling it all for you."

"But he gets online…"

"To play Solitaire," I said. "And he's not even really playing Solitaire. He just thinks he is."

With Daddy's last fall in the kitchen, Mom had really lost everything. Before, even though she had to have known she was losing it, she had still pretended she knew all about her finances and insurances and bills, and when Michelle or I had asked, she had become indignant. Although she had no idea what day it was, even back in January of 2016, she had been pretending she knew what was going on and hadn't dared let her daughters or anyone else know otherwise. Having some measure of control in her life while her mind ran wild had become the one thing she had to hold on to and I had finally understood that.

Okay, so, full disclosure. This is the point where I really piled on a resident, but I figured he would never know and Mom needed the boost. *Operation Dignity for Momma* must be played. When I told Michelle about the "you have the power" conversation with Mom, Michelle agreed it was perfect. Together, we decided it was crucial for Mom to believe she held all the cards. We convinced Mom that she—Mom—was the key to everyone not killing Daddy, that she—Mom—was so darned lovable that she—Mom—kept people from disliking Daddy. That was why she was living in the facility. We needed her to keep an eye on things. We insisted that was why Daddy needed her. *Everyone* needed Mom. She was vital to all of it.

Still, she's not an idiot.

As Daddy paced the halls at odd hours, punching Kimberly and stealing other people's clothing, he didn't exactly wow people with his diplomacy.

Our entire childhood, our father had a crew cut. Even when he began doing intelligence work and let the short buzz gain some length, he was never shaggy or unkempt. He was never disheveled or out of order. Neat. Trim. Muscular. Athletic. The White Knight was a spit-shine example of discipline and control. Now, however, he sometimes sported women's clothing, usually Mom's, and wore multiple layers for reasons we couldn't understand.

On a day Kerri and Katie came by to visit, Daddy was wearing one slipper, one running shoe, Mom's pants, three shirts, and one of Mom's necklaces.

While Kerri was alarmed and saddened, Katie broke into a smile and checked him out, head to toe.

"What, uh…" Katie wagged a finger at his outfit. "What'cha got goin' on here, Papa?"

The girls did not see our parents as often as Michelle and I and weren't privy to the varied fashion statements Daddy, aka Papa, had picked up. Marc Powe lived in the world of what's-yours-is-mine and what's-mine-is-mine. He put on whatever he wanted from whomever he wanted.

So, to all the family members of the residents our father was taking clothing from: We know this was happening and are sorry. We try to return things. We try to ensure that he only wear his own clothing, but he's a freaking super spy! We can't stop him!

Instead—and this is where *Operation Dignity for Momma* and the open apology to extended family members of residents comes in—I've been throwing other residents under the proverbial bus for a while now.

Sorry.

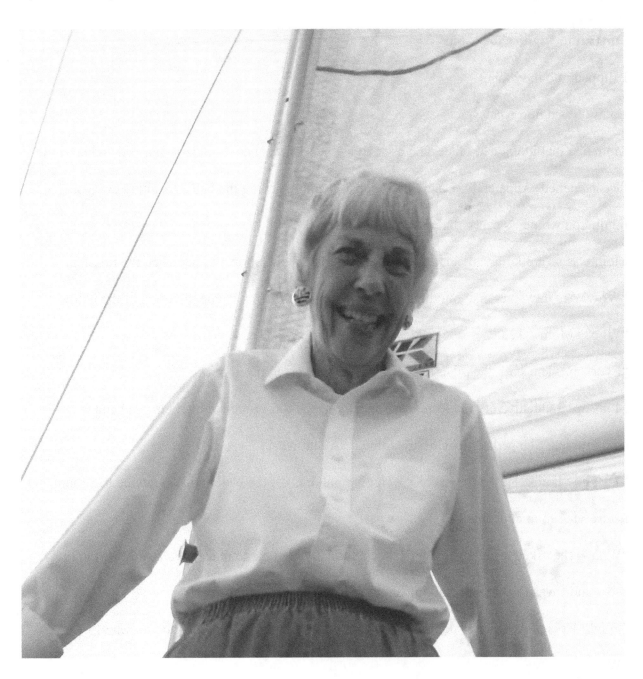

Patricia Caston, aka to all as Ms. Pat, on a sailboat, yet this is the perfect picture as she towered over us all—literally and figuratively

Operation Dignity for Mom

I slipped into the room.

Daddy was doing whatever.

Mom had that look on her face, and as soon as she saw me, her shoulders slumped and her little face saddened. Apparently, Daddy had been at it again, pacing the halls, irritating everyone, putting on women's pants, and refusing directives.

Mom was so embarrassed, and I gave an exaggerated exhalation and launched the mission.

"Wow! Are they ever mad out there!" I pointed my thumb in a vague direction of the hallway.

"Who?" Mom asked.

"Everyone. The staff, the other residents…everyone is talking about it."

Mom was suddenly very interested and better yet, she'd forgotten about being sad and embarrassed. She perked up. Gossip loomed. "About what?"

"That guy Frank. He's a maniac. He's ripping pictures off the wall and flooded the bathroom and is throwing food at people!"

"Who?" she asked again and even flashed a little double take to make sure Daddy was in the room and I wasn't somehow talking about him.

"Frank! He's one of the residents and they are pretty danged hot, let me tell you what!"

"Who?"

Mom didn't know names of anyone and had a hard time keeping up with who is who. I used this to my advantage.

"The staff. They can't stand him!" I waved my hands at her like, *C'mon, don't you know? It's Frank. EVERYONE hates Frank!* For added effect, "He's such an ass!" *Sorry, Frank.*

Over the course of the next couple of weeks, Michelle joined in and *Operation Dignity for Momma* became a hugely successful campaign as we continued to throw a few more residents under the proverbial memory-care bus. As far as Mom knew, Daddy was awesome compared to some of the residents, especially Frank, and on the days the staff might seem a little short or impatient with Daddy, well, that was only be because that damned Frank broke the refrigerator or ruined lunch.

Was it too hot in the building? *Frank!*

The TV wasn't working? *Frank.*

Daddy went into someone room and messed up their bed? *Frank*!

Operation Dignity for Momma restored more power to our Mom and just in time, as more things were slipping away. She may not have known where her underwear was, but she knew that Frank was a damned idiot.

Chapter Eleven

FACEBOOK: *May 2017*

> *The most amazing gift...*
> *We had a yard sale at my parents' house and sold many things that were hard to part with, but it had to be done. Because of my dad's job, there were TONS of things from Iraq, all over Africa, Middle East, Russia, Germany, etc. Some we knew the history if, but most we did not.*
> *We sold a cool looking plaque, clearly Arabic, and figured the inscription meant, "Go in peace," "Blessings upon you," or something else common to the region.*
> *Michelle ended up with a young man knocking on her door. He'd bought the plaque a year ago.*
> *He told her that his brother was a linguist and the words spelled out our father's name and they used that to look our father up online. "Your father is a very highly decorated officer."*
> *When the young man learned our father's history, his reputation in the intelligence world, he knew he had to return the plaque to us. He even refused to be reimbursed.*
> *To this man who found us...thank you doesn't cover it.*
> *What a beautiful, beautiful gift. THANK YOU...*
> *Blessings upon you!*

Communication is life.

I know. It sounds like a bit of an overstatement.

It's not.

Communication is a life skill that allows us to connect, relate, empathize, and realize. Through communication, we build trust, respect, and relationships. We solve problems, make connections, develop businesses, and create entire communities. Communication allows for greater love, affection, better care, bigger ideas, and, in the case of our father, save a life. Daddy's skill as a communicator was one of the things that made him one of the most recognized and decorated military attachés to serve our nation. So, when I was assigned the task of writing a book about successful entrepreneurs, it was only natural I interview my father. It was the year 2000, and he had retired from the U.S. military and moved into the private sector as head of security for World Bank, United Nations, and UNICEF. He was big doins' in the security world.

He taught me the nuances of networking, from being mindful when using a network to benefiting others while maintaining a good standing to understanding the importance of being generous, "because it is the natural thing to do." He received so much because he gave so much more.

Sometimes, it was hard to remember how it once was with him as we struggled with yet another memory-care facility.

After a few months in the new location, now his sixth move, Daddy was completely non-verbal. Most days, he didn't recognize Michelle or me and had this distant, detached look in his eyes that made it clear there was no hope of any return. Our dad was gone. Worse, he was angry. He was acting out, and where some of his antics had been amusing before, this man was not funny. He was urinating in other people's rooms...on their floors. He was fighting with the staff and upsetting Mom so horribly that she, too, had no other place to go but downhill. Fast.

During one visit, Michelle and I noted several things. The other residents were zonked out of their heads. No one walked around. No one talked. They were just zombie bodies, strewn about, in recliner chairs. And the staff had little interaction with the residents. The few staff members we did like didn't stay long. Clearly, they were unhappy in their jobs, and it was reflected in the care and cleanliness of the facility.

To make matters worse, Mom and Daddy's room flooded repeatedly.

The first two times, we were told it was Daddy's fault, and briefly, we accepted it as gospel. I mean, why not? He was doing everything else wrong. But after two more times, when the width of the flooding extended to either side of our parents' king-sized bed, it did not seem humanly possible for him to access that much water.

Michelle and I were also distracted and baffled by the fact that not one, not two, but *three* expensive king-sized waterproof mattress covers had simply disappeared. Given our parents were the *only* couple with a king-sized bed, it seemed odd. More than odd, it seemed criminal. With each disappearance, Michelle and I turned the place upside down (without much help from the staff), looking in the laundry room, kitchen, storages areas, each resident's room, closets, under beds, and in the common area. Three king-sized mattress covers, all gone without explanation.

Hmmm.

The flooding continued as our parents, now without any of the mattress covers we had specifically bought for them to protect both their own skin and the mattress, began soiling the bed.

It wasn't long before our parents contracted scabies—a contagious, intensely itchy skin condition caused by a tiny, burrowing mite.

According to the Centers for Disease Control and Prevention, nursing homes are highly susceptible to scabies and, no surprise, urine-soaked mattresses make excellent breeding grounds for the mites.

Without calling to tell us what was going on, the staff then quarantined our parents to their room to prevent the scabies from spreading.

Michelle and I found them in their room—Daddy seated in his chair, with his faraway look, but Mom was miserable, holding a paper plate of food, and fidgeting.

"What are you doing?" I asked her.

"Oh!" She looked so relieved to see us. She told us "those women" were making her stand in one place to eat her food.

Initially, we laughed. It sounded absurd, and she was prone to less-than-accurate remarks.

But, it turned out Mom wasn't too far off the mark.

The staff had carried her food into her room along with an order to "stay here."

Mom took that to mean, in the very spot she was standing when she was handed the food. She, an itty-bitty ninety-pound woman, had been standing in that very spot, afraid to move, ever since.

We sat her on the bed and began talking when I was overwhelmed.

I looked at Michelle. "Man, I am itching all over!"

Michelle was too.

We both looked at the bed.

A visiting nurse later advised us to call the state on the facility.

We bought a new bed, set up delivery, and wrestled with what to do about calling the state. I cannot emphasize enough how frightened we were that our parents would be punished if we complained.

The next day, I was under Mom's bed, searching for a missing shoe, when I pulled out a boot soaked with water.

I pushed the bed to the side and, lo and behold, water was seeping up in an area no larger than a shoebox. I had inadvertently discovered the source before it spread—again.

I found a staff member who confided that another room had flooded as well.

Soon, however, that claim was wildly disputed, and the manager insisted that our father, with his oh-so-speedy, turbo-turtle shuffle, was collecting large cups of water, getting down on his hands and knees, and then crawling partway under the bed to, with precision aim, throw the water precisely onto the floor in the dead center of the king-sized bed.

Ah. Yes. Well. That does make sense. I stared at her. "You're not serious."

But she was.

Two days later, the fire department was called out as the water pipe burst, and all the residents were forced to move to another building for the night.

Wow. My dad can sure throw the water around....

My rage was quietly building again. It was bad enough that we had been ripped off so many times in the beginning but now, at the tune of nine thousand dollars a month, our parents were eating off paper plates, using plastic forks with every meal, having personal items stolen, soiling their unprotected bed, and contracting scabies.

As a result, we were forced to 1) move our parents to another room only to be told that we would have to pay for the installation of a new TV in the new location, and 2) that all of this was still my father's fault. Additionally, despite paying for our father to receive the *Dallas Morning News* in hopes he would read the headlines out loud as he once had, no one could recall the last time they had seen a newspaper in our parents' room.

Still, I told Michelle we couldn't move them again. We just couldn't. Daddy needed to find his footing, literally and figuratively. I was so terrified of his regressing even further that I stupidly, blindly fought to keep him in that hellhole.

Then, they acquired a second round of scabies.

Another visiting nurse was appalled by our parents' treatment and pulled Michelle to the side. She said we had to get our parents out and get them out F-A-S-T.

What choice did we have? Yet, how did we know wherever we went next wouldn't be just as bad?

I, the Peter Pan of our family, the eternal optimist, the one nicknamed Evergreen, no longer had faith in the system or with any caregivers. I'd reached a new level of frustration. When people learned about Mom and Daddy and tried to empathize, I couldn't work up the energy to care. One parent or grandparent going "through it," while the rest of the family stood strong, is not the same.

You're feeling a fractured toe, but we actually have a shattered femur. Not the same. *Your canoe, just off the shoreline, has a slow leak. Our ship, the* Titanic, *is going down in the middle of the ocean, with no land in sight, and I just spotted a group of man-eating sharks circling.*

As you can see, I was very busy planning an upcoming pity party.

On the day Michelle and I tag-teamed Mom and Daddy for a doctor's appointment to assess their medical condition and the extent of their scabies before they could be moved again, Nationwide Pet Insurance and First American Home Warranty were both still trying to collect money from my parents while refusing to answer their own business phones.

The pet insurance had been withdrawing sixty dollars a month for a dog that died eight years prior!

I really wasn't in the mood to wrestle in a parking lot.

Daddy's always on a timeline, so once the doctor was done with him, I wheeled him out to the car while Michelle finished up with Mom. We didn't dare stay inside with Daddy already eyeing the fire alarm and ready to bolt.

Besides, I was still privately planning my pity party. *Hmm. What do I need? I'll need some more misery, perhaps another bank scare, and—*

As I wheeled Daddy to the car, hoping to get him inside without incident, I heard, "Oooookay."

Shit.

"I'm really not in the mood to wrestle in the parking lot. Come on, Daddy, just put your leg into—"

He set his jaw and it was on like Donkey Kong.

I tried everything. Duck and bob and weave. "I'VE GOT JAZZ HANDS!" Knowing Michelle was just inside the office, I called her cell—one handed—while I waved a single jazz hand at Daddy.

She ran outside, leaving Mom (always a gamble) with the doctor, and together we tried physically placing our father into the car. How to put another human being, who is freakishly strong, into a car without hurting him?

"JUST BEND YOUR KNEE, DADDY! BEEEENNND!"

Michelle had a solid half-nelson grip around his shoulders while I crouched low, applying soft elbow strikes to the back of his knee.

Whack, whack, whack.

"Just [gasp] bend [wheeze] your [ugh]…how the hell are [more gasping] you this [grunt] this freaking [pant, pant] strong?"

Whack, whack, whack.

A car slowly rolled by.

I realized what we must look like and burst out laughing. The gawking driver probably thought we were mugging this poor senior citizen.

Suddenly, Michelle and I were both laughing so hard, we couldn't move.

As we rolled and struggled to breathe between giggles, Daddy joined in. And only because we got him laughing did we manage to get him into the car.

Michelle ran back in to be with Mom while I, now hot and sweaty, buckled in beside Daddy and said, "Ooooooookay."

In 1985, following Daddy's "arrest" by the Kuwait government, Iraq literally gave my parents twenty-four hours to leave the country, so we had them come stay with us. After their immediate expulsion from Baghdad, Mom, Daddy, and our grandmother, came to live with me, Michelle, and our two roommates, outside D.C. They were dark times for our dad as the White House, Pentagon, DIA, and CIA sorted out the details of the surveillance, imprisonment (or detainment, depending on which side you're on), and release of one of their military attachés.

U.S. News and World Report ran a small but powerful article entitled, "An American Spy in Kuwait." For our father, it was an embarrassment made worse when he was later told to just *hang out*. Marc Powe isn't a hang out kind of guy. He wanted to be in on the action, back at work, and proactive.

I decided to bring him a little cheer by telling him about my college communications course assignment, which required reporting on the country of Jordon as though I was a citizen. Queen Noor actually was an American citizen and, in my naive mind, it stood to reason I would just call her up and talk to her.

I was twenty years old. What do you expect?

Daddy was aghast. "Don't be absurd!" he warned me, barely looking up from his newspaper.

"You can't just call the queen and ask how the weather is."

I called the operator and was connected to the international operator.

I asked to speak with the operator of Jordan and heard my father chuckle.

"It's ringing," I reported, holding a hand over the receiver.

My father raised an eyebrow.

I asked to speak to the palace operator because, well, that seemed the next place to go, right? Daddy snorted behind his newspaper. Colonel Marc Powe was a man of precision and decision. There was protocol to be followed at all times. There were rules and regulations; a certain law and order required. There were certain, reliable, pre-determined ways in which a person was to operate. One did not simply pick up a phone and ask to speak to the palace operator and expect to—

"It's ringing," I whispered, and he lowered his newspaper.

When a far-away voice answered in Arabic, I asked to speak to someone who spoke English.

"It's ringing," I said again, and I sensed my father sit forward a bit. Half a smile formed as I asked if I might speak to the Queen. "It's ringing."

By now, my father had abandoned his newspaper, and a full-blown smile covered his face. It was nice to see because he hadn't been doing a lot of smiling lately.

His smile, however, was quickly replaced with utter dismay when I asked to speak to the Queen's assistant. *Seriously, what else do you call a person who might assist a Queen in her Queenly duties?* I made my way past another English-speaking person and then to the Queen's personal secretary.

The man who had seen and heard it all could do nothing more than shake his head as I eventually got my shot at speaking with Queen Noor and…panicked. I actually asked her how the weather was in Jordan.

During the same timeframe, a huge snowstorm blew through Northern Virginia and Washington D.C., and my little car ended up buried in snow.

Ever determined to get to work, despite warnings from my father and city officials, I headed outside to dig my car out.

Frustrated but also happy to have something to do, Daddy began shoveling with me while also giving his brand of sage advice regarding weather conditions, work ethic, and my shoveling methods.

At some point, his lecture grew tiresome, and I made some snarky comment about him not understanding my confinement.

There are very few times in my life that my dad has ever raised his voice at me, *very* few. But this was one of those times and it was a doozey.

"I don't understand?!" He was incredulous. He railed about how I would never understand being confined in a cell, a prisoner…in the dark.

Honestly, I know there was more, but I was so stunned, then angry—angry about what happened to him, about us being packed into our small house, like cord wood, about him not being there when I needed him…and I came right back at him. "Yeah? Well maybe I understand all too well, and maybe *you* have no idea what it's like to be a victim of a violent crime!"

Daddy froze.

We found we had both been victims of something we really couldn't share with other people. We had been treated in a way that there were no take-backs, no undoing, and no forgetting.

Like my father, I speak very sparingly of those days, but I will say this—after our stunning announcements, we nodded at each other, kind of laughed, in a shared but sorrowful way, and went back to shoveling mounds and mounds of snow.

Thirty-one years later, sitting in the car together, waiting for Michelle and Mom to finish with the doctor, I zipped over to Sonic's drive-thru and ordered him a coffee.

Content with his drink, he relaxed, and I found NPR on the radio. We both settled in and drove around for a while.

With Mom in the car, I always feel the need to talk as she is so lonely and afraid. With Daddy, no words are needed.

During a commercial break, I said, "Let's call someone!"

As it happened, I didn't even need to dream up someone as an earth-bound angel had already picked up a phone and was calling me—Mari Grace. She's a nurse at a facility we were hoping to move to as soon as we got the medical paperwork completed with our doctor. She was having a difficult time deciphering our parents' medical records from the memory-care facility they were currently in.

Even as I heard myself relaying story after story, I realized how wrong it all was. It really hit me just how much we had allowed ourselves to be bullied by health-care providers in charge of our parents' lives. I couldn't even answer Mari Grace's questions about what my parents were ingesting in the way of medication. I had no idea. *Wait a minute! Aren't we in charge? Don't I have Power of Attorney?*

A family should be entitled to know what is happening with their loved one. Yet, the memory-care facility never gave us straight answers about our parents' medication, how much or what they were being given. We didn't even understand how the pharmacy worked.

Mari Grace asked more questions, and I listened as I kept repeating, "I don't know," over and over again. Not two months prior, Daddy had fallen again and had been transported to the local hospital. He had required seven staples in his head but had been immediately released to return to the memory-care facility.

If you're keeping track, this marks his eleventh significant hit to the head. Because of his condition, Daddy doesn't know how to bring his hands up to protect himself in a fall like other people do instinctively. Instead, with hands at his sides, his head always makes full contact with the floor.

A month later, Michelle inquired about the staples.

What staples?

"You know, the staples that were put in his head after he fell."

Here's where it gets good.

The staff, despite an ambulance arriving to retrieve our father and subsequent medical report, despite his being admitted into the ER and receiving medical treatment, despite a late-night call informing us of our father's 1) fall and 2) staples as treatment for an open head wound following said fall, we were informed by the facility that there had been no fall, ergo, no staples.

This was who and what we were dealing with.

We couldn't move fast enough, and I dearly wished I had done so earlier.

As the paperwork was finalized, the owner of the memory-care facility, still fully blaming our father for the flooding, the scabies, the theft/loss, and the neglect by offering "your father is a very difficult man" as the reason why, called me as soon as he learned we were taking our nine thousand dollars a month somewhere else.

It is important to note, when I discovered my parents had been blamed for "losing" their mattress covers and I called the owner to ask for some help, he never called back. When fecal matter sat on a wooden chair in my parents' room for six straight days and I called to ask for assistance, he never called back. When Michelle called following an incident with the flooding and concern over medications, he never called back. When unexplained bruises appeared on my father's body and Michelle took pictures and called, he never called back.

Yet, the moment we were prepared to move our parents—devastated and defeated by terrible treatment and the repeated displays of unprofessionalism, I got a call.

It is also important to note this same owner was known for showing up—uninvited—to open-house career days for caregivers at another large, more upscale memory-care facility to recruit potential employees for his own organization. Simply put, well after doing business with this person, Michelle and I learned how truly unsatisfactory many things were about him and his business practices.

Later, when I learned that a health-care placement center was still recommending this facility to families, I told the agent about our horrendous experience in the hope of preventing the same things happening to another family.

This is one of those agencies that promises to find a home for your mom (or dad) and promotes itself as an unbiased agency. Instead, it is paid by those institutions to recommend them. I appreciate capitalism as much as the next guy, but no one deserves to be treated this way.

I wanted the agency promising great care to know who and what they were endorsing. Because her agency received a cut each time a family was placed with a company/memory-care facility, the agent was unwilling to hear the truth.

The importance of effective networking and communication cannot be emphasized enough, particularly when we are talking about memory and long-term care for those who cannot defend themselves.

The phone rang, and caller ID prepared me for what was coming. Or, so I thought.

The owner asked why we were leaving and actually said, "I think we can agree that the care your parents have received has been exceptional."

I was never combative. I was never unkind. I never raised my voice. Quite the opposite. I was very quiet as I told him about the flooding, the scabies, the bruises, the ongoing questions about medication, proper grooming, and cleanliness for our parents.

"But we know for a fact that your father was flooding the room, and your father got scabies from the hospital."

It was clear he and his staff would never own up to anything. The company, as a whole, were determined to stick by what sounded good to them, and so I simply said nothing while he tried to persuade us not to leave. The loss of our nine grand a month was significant, I knew, since several more vacancies had opened up at that facility as well. I was unmoved. I knew too much and there was no going back.

And that was when he went low. "I would hate to see you burn a bridge. In three days, your father is going to get kicked out of the new place, and then where will you go?"

It was a low blow. Still, I didn't say a word, and he gave a nervous laugh.

"Of course, we would always take you back, but why put your father through another move?"

I hung up the phone and began shaking. My dad had not been easy throughout any of this, but he's a good man—a great man—and he deserved so much better than what he had been getting. I just had to believe there was still hope out there. I wanted to find a place where he would be treated with respect and love and kindness. Was that so much to ask?

Gawd!

This was made even more frustrating because my dad was exactly the person I would have called for advice.

Ironically, I found my old business-entrepreneur interview with Daddy in one of my books.

We had talked about the importance of networking, and he'd remarked that, whether talking to a business leader, sports agent, writer, or peacekeeper, the philosophy was always the same. "You always try to build a relationship, try to establish some common interest, and follow up quickly with an email or phone call. If you are truly a good networker, you can't be selfish. You have to be willing to give to people. My philosophy for good networking comes into play by ending phone calls with the question, 'Is there anything else I can do for you?' It's a sincere question, but it will also engender people to being helpful in return."

My dad, the genius.

Thanks, Daddy.

And so, I picked up the phone and called the office of Isle at Watercrest.

Chapter Twelve

FACEBOOK: *April 2017*

> *A day in the life of memory care:*
> *Hit someone super early in the morning then eat a big breakfast with them, dance, and take a nap.*
> *I know it sounds like an episode from* Keeping up with the Kardashians *but this is Keepin' Up with Marc Powe.*

On February 10th, exactly thirty-four days after moving my parents into Isle at Watercrest and thirty-six days after being warned by the other care facility owner my father would be kicked to the curb in mere days, and after almost ten months of only saying (for the most part) "okay" and "well," Daddy spoke a full sentence to me and Kerri.

We had all become used to no eye contact or any assurances that he knew who we were. Talking *at* him rather than *to* him, however unintentional, had become our main form of communication. You can imagine our shock, after months of nothing but Daddy's rumored reign of terror from the other facility's staff, when he stood up, swept his hand outward in a grand gesture, and asked Kerri and me, "Would you like some coffee?"

She and I stared at each other for several seconds before Kerri, a non-coffee drinker, laughed out loud and said, "Yes!"

Too late. Daddy had already walked away. But still!

The journey we have taken to get to this place has been beyond hard, beyond unfair, beyond unhealthy, and downright wrong. We have filed a formal complaint with the state about the lack of care provided by the previous facility upon the recommendations of more than a dozen other caregivers and health professionals. Still, they remain very much in business.

We've learned all about overmedicating and heavily sedating residents in memory-care facilities is extremely common so the "caregivers" don't have to deal with active old people. For a man like Marc Powe, however, who cannot be kept down, translates into multiple falls. Again and again and again he fell because, while over-medicated, he could not quite get his bearings as he negotiated the halls at 2 and 3 o'clock in the morning.

Since arriving at Isle of Watercrest, there have been no falls and, interestingly enough, no odd early morning wandering.

How was that possible?

"He's happier," one caregiver said, matter-of-factly. No sarcastic or snarky commentary against the former facility, just a simple statement she knew to be true.

Happier also meant regaining a kind of trust Michelle and I hadn't fully realized was lost.

One day, quite innocently, Maria (an awesome angel placed here to care for those who cannot care for themselves) and Norma (another awesome angel placed here to care for those who cannot care for themselves) were explaining how they had worked with our father to help him overcome his fear of the shower.

Since when is he afraid of the shower?

It was clear to them that he had been forced to take cold showers and, as a result, was scared of showering. They had seen this type of behavior before and they'd recognized it for what it was.

He had, presumably, learned those who showered him were the enemy.

Oh, my God. I mean…we'd suspected it. We had worried and stressed about it but…

How many times had Mom told us about cold showers, but we hadn't believed her? What kind of sick person forces naked, scared, elderly people, with varying forms of dementia, into cold showers? We just couldn't believe it and so…we hadn't.

Until now.

Norma and Maria described spending large amounts of time standing next to a running shower so our dad could touch the water on his own terms and feel for himself that it was nice and warm. They explained how the act of stepping into the shower had to be *his* idea—he taking a shower rather than have one forced upon him. They wanted him to remember and know a shower could be a pleasant experience.

That Michelle and I were excited about our parents eating off real plates, with real silverware, was, I know, pathetic, but we were over the moon. That we continued to be surprised by updates on our parents or gleefully discovering (and sharing with others) Isle at Watercrest had an event coordinator "who actually does stuff with the residents!" was probably more sad than anything else, but the past year's lack of care and concern for seniors at every facility we'd inhabited and/or frequented had numbed us. We weren't expecting anything better.

We had gone from *nothing but the best for our parents* to *could you just kind of watch them and make sure he doesn't fall*, forgetting to ask *could you please not hit him in the process?*

I stepped into Isle at Watercrest to find Mari Grace waiting.

She wanted to talk about the amount of medication my parents were on. Specifically, she was startled by how much they had been given and wondered why.

I had no answer.

But we both knew.

Still, she just wanted assurances I had not encouraged that level of medication. She wanted me to know that there, at the Isle, they wanted their residents on as few medications as possible; they wanted their residents coherent and active; they liked their residents to be mobile and walking the halls and being social.

I extended my arm toward her. "Pinch me." *No seriously!* I felt as though I was in heaven. This was all we ever wanted for our parents.

Even now, I cannot help thinking of all the seniors we left behind from all the other places and I am so sorry because I wish they could be here, at the Isle, too. This is how our seniors should be care for. This is how all humans should be cared for.

Every morning, Londa, a lovely loud, hilarious, vivacious events coordinator for Isle at Watercrest, says the Pledge of Allegiance with her residents.

While Daddy was still adjusting—his sleeping patterns were a bit off to start—he missed these morning events. One morning, however, he happened to be up and eating in the dining hall when he heard the pledge being recited in the next room.

The caregivers and Londa reported he'd nearly toppled a chair trying to get to the common room and pledge his own allegiance.

And that's just one example! The stories are nonstop now, as are the video images sent to me and Michelle. The difference is as if everything prior was in black and white—we either knew too much too late or knew nothing at all. Since entering the doors of the Isle, everything has color again. They are the gold at the end of the rainbow!

The point here is not to sing Isle's praises so much as serve a reminder to you, the reader, that this should be the norm. This is the kind of care we *should* expect for our loved ones and these examples are meant to provide guidelines for you when you are searching for a memory-care facility.

During Mardi Gras week, we received a video of Mom dancing and twirling an umbrella while many of the caregivers encouraged her every step.

"Work it, Ms. Karen! Work it, girl!"

Oh, how I laughed. Mom *was* workin' it!

Still, through no fault of the facility, no place is perfect. Mom's changing personality and personal war with a progressive disease is a game-changer.

By moving Mom into a facility that placed her on fewer medication, she was suddenly more cognizant of her living situation. Sadly, she frequently said, "This isn't how I imagined my life." It was agonizing. It broke our hearts over and over as her clarity also allowed her to recognize what she had lost and was still losing in her life. Yet, within that same moment of great revelation, she would lean in and tell us about Daddy going back to work or leaving her for one of the girls or report Daddy saying horrible things to her. Moreover, we know she prowls her room in the wee hours of the night and early morning, trying to wake Daddy or neurotically hide things as she's sure people are stealing from her.

Which would explain why Michelle and I find Daddy's socks, her underwear, and puzzle pieces in the weirdest places!

Because Mom cannot remember that Daddy is brain damaged and because, after all the trauma, Daddy thinks very little about his wife, if at all, she is determined he is having affairs with several of the women at the Isle. In fact, this has been an ongoing fear of hers since he became incapacitated and her paranoia ramped up, but the Isle has made it worse because 1) she is less medicated, and 2) Daddy is happier.

Picture this:

Alex: Hey, Momma! How's it going?

Mom: Oh, there you are! Those girls are all over your father!

Alex: What? What girls? (Internally, I cringe. I know what she means by the *girls,* but hope springs eternal, and I pretend maybe a fleet of Girl Scouts just arrived and are working on merit badges for senior-care giving, or maybe a lost band of small wandering children—all girls—are in need of terrific navigational skills and happened upon my father because he used to have a great sense of direction).

Mom: You know! The ones who are always here, giggling, and constantly pawing at your father!

Alex: Well, I don't think they're paw—

Mom: They are! They are always running in here, day and night, and ripping off his clothes.

Alex: Well, Mom, they are only changing his clothes for the day. (I'm fairly certain they aren't giggling either, but I let that part slide).

Mom: They are not! They are pulling off his pants and…

Alex: Okay, *ew*! Mom. Stop. I swear to you…I *promise*, they are *only* doing their jobs, and they are changing his clothes for the day so that he can be fresh and clean.

Mom: Their hands are all over him. And they dig in his pockets and take all his money.

Alex: Mom! He doesn't have any money.

Mom: (She considers this for a moment and then shrugs.)

Alex: Let's go find him, talk to him, and you can see no one is hanging all over him. (Before we make it two feet, I see Daddy and Thelma, a very pretty Nigerian caregiver—this is relevant because Daddy loves Nigerians—stroll by, arm in arm, laughing. *Ugh.*

Mom: See?!

Another day, while she's explaining to me why we need to "get out," she points to Trent, an extremely sweet man and fairly new resident. "See that man?"

I nod. "Trent? He's awesome. I love Trent." And I do. I try to talk to him every time I see him. At the time, Trent had a hair brush in one pocket and an electric razor, which I admit, looked like Daddy's, in the other pocket.

"That man steals from everyone!" Mom says.

Yes. Well.

Our die-hard, through-and-through old Ag father, a member of the Corps of Cadets, graduate of Texas A&M University, and hater of all things Texas Longhorn is in possession of a Longhorn ball cap. This would be the same ball cap that hangs neatly beside a U.S. Navy cap. Our father is Army all the way. We are also in possession of an Alabama sweatshirt, which I don't understand, but have learned to stop asking too many questions.

"He goes into everyone's rooms and just takes whatever he wants!" As Mom regales me with the adventures of Trent, Daddy sit down beside me.

I look at his arm and ask Mom, "Whose watch is that on Daddy's arm?"

Mercifully, for Mom, it doesn't count when Daddy ransacks and pillages the town, and so we mostly talk about what a thief Trent is.

Trent's cool. I like Trent. Secretly, I hope to encourage his nefarious exploits through the halls of the Isle because it gives Mom something to obsess over other than Daddy. And that's the point of all this. Mom is now just coherent enough to care more about her surroundings, and it is hard on all of us.

For the past seven months, Michelle and/or I have taken Mom out several times a week. We've gone on short shopping trips, to lunch, gotten ice cream, gone to the park, or sometimes just driven around. It has been important to get Mom out of whatever facility we've been in, not only for her own piece of mind, but Daddy's as well. She never lets him be. She always fussed with or around him because she honestly cannot remember what's going on with him. For her, her brilliant and always charming husband is suddenly cold and very distant. For a time, she seemed to have greater clarity when she was outside with one of us, hence the trips.

Many of our outings are highly comical; most are eye-openers.

Mom has no idea how to eat certain foods anymore.

The first time I noticed it, she asked for a Coney hot dog. I watched in disbelief as she tried to eat it upside down, not understanding how and why the toppings kept falling in her lap. Next, it was a cupcake. Then, a slice of pizza. If we drove through Starbucks, I couldn't allow Mom access to coffee because she kept trying to take the lid off and would invariably burn her hand.

I called Michelle in distress only to learn Michelle had experienced similar issues with a sandwich, a brownie, and a pastry.

It wasn't just food. She no longer understood how straws worked or seatbelts and had no idea how to put on her own jacket, coat, or sweater. In fact, there were times both of us would be laughing as she twirled around and around, losing her tiny self in a sea of fabric until I would call her out. "You're doing this on purpose!"

But one day, when she was crying—and she frequently cries—I asked, "What's wrong?" Again, this was such a stupid question to ask a person losing everything she had ever known, but what else was I supposed to do?

"I can't tell you."

"Why?" I wanted to know.

"Because this isn't the kind of thing a mother should share with her child."

She was so sad, and I said that, while we were mother/daughter, we were also friends, and I wanted her to talk to me as a friend. While the details are unimportant, she admitted Daddy hurt her feelings because he was uninterested in her. She had initiated intimate relations with him and had been—she felt—spurned.

For months, I had been securing her seatbelt, directing her where to walk and sit, opening doors, assisting with straws, and cutting up food. I tied her shoes, helped her in the bathroom, and got her arms through the sleeves of countless jackets and sweaters, but this?

A sigh so heavy it could not be contained slipped out of me, and Mom slumped in her seat.

"Mom, no man has ever loved his wife more than Daddy has loved you."

It's true. And perhaps, it was what made all of this so tragic. My father, to his own detriment, demise, and self-torture at times, loved my mother beyond compare. He denied her nothing.

Despite all the years of hard work and strife it took to achieve an unparalleled career in the Army, all while maintaining a reputation beyond reproach, our father never became a general, and we knew it was because of our mother. She betrayed him, yet he never left her side. She was unconventional, never fully capable of playing the role of military wife, yet he never complained. He never yelled at her—not once.

Every Wednesday, for more than a decade, he brought home flowers for his wife. And when her mind began to go, he made excuses and assured no one ever knew she had lost even one step. He cherished and worshiped and spoiled. I wanted to cry.

She had lost so much more than I'd realized.

"Mom, he just doesn't understand things like sex anymore." It was little comfort, but it was all I had to offer.

What made it worse was that Daddy no longer understood *love* the way he once had.

Michelle and I were losing our dad, but Mom was losing her soul mate, while he was standing right beside her.

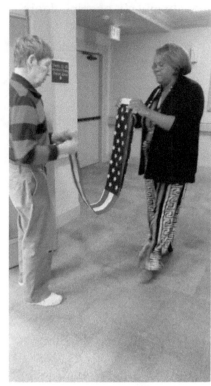

Londa Gittens, events coordinator and director at Isle of Watercrest, figuring out how much the flag means to him, always plays the National Anthem and lets him fold the flag with her.

Despite his dementia and brain damage...the Colonel STILL recognizes his beloved flag!

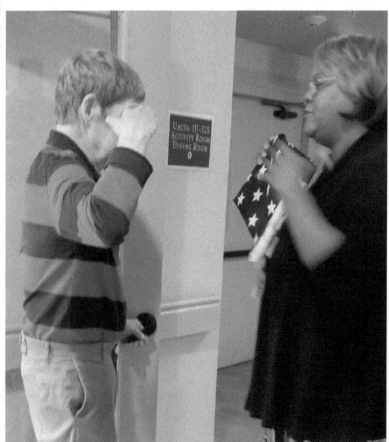

Chapter Thirteen

FACEBOOK: *March 2017*

> *If you've ever wondered how a criminal trespasser justifies his/her crime, let me help you out:*
> *My dad wandered into another resident's room at 6 am.*
> *Resident protests, calls for help, caregiver arrives, and my dad and the caregiver begin to wrestle then…MOM jumps into the fight to "help."*
> *What?*
> *She weighs ninety-two pounds, soaking wet! And how does she figure Daddy needs help…assaulting the caregiver AND trespassing?*
> *Alex: Mom! You can't encourage Daddy to go in other people's rooms. Why did you turn on the caregiver? Why not help her get Daddy out? That wasn't your room.*
> *Mom's comeback was something she always told me when I was growing up—Don't start a fight, but always finish it.*
> *Well, okay.*
> *Mom: They're sorry they messed with us.*
> *I'm thinking about starting a new hashtag—#DementiaOnlyBothersThoseWithoutIt*

On December 9th, 1961, our father married a woman who had been raised in country clubs where most—okay, let's be honest, *all*—work had been done for her. She had no clue what to do with a stove. She had no idea how to make coffee, boil an egg, or even make toast.

As a newly married couple, our parents rented a small apartment attached to a larger home. Daddy was just beginning his career in the military, and Mom was trying her hand at cooking. Every morning, she made her new husband a cup of coffee, eggs, and homemade biscuits. Life was reportedly good.

After a time, however, the homeowners got curious about the throngs of birds converging on their garage, so they climbed to the second level to get a better look. Dozens of mini white discs scattered across the roof seemed to have piqued the birds' interest. Still, the homeowners had no idea what the objects were.

When our father returned from work one day, the male homeowner asked if Daddy had any idea what was on the rooftop.

The then-young Captain Powe flushed, embarrassed. He knew.

Each morning, he'd claimed he was in a rush and gathered up the "yummy" biscuits "for the road." As he had gotten into his car, he'd chucked them over his shoulder. He had been throwing the inedible biscuits his new bride had made on top of the garage for weeks. His hope had been that the birds would disappear, taking the biscuits with them, but not even the birds had wanted the unappetizing white hockey pucks once they'd tried a bite or two. He begged the homeowner not to tell and promised he would remove the biscuits that weekend, but before he could, Mom found out.

The homeowner's wife took pity on Mom and began giving her cooking lessons.

Many, many years later, I asked Daddy how long he figured he could have gotten away that charade, and he said he'd still be doing it today if the birds had only cooperated.

Through thick and thin, hard times and inedible biscuits, he was committed.

This past December marked fifty-five years of marriage, but it was the first time our father wasn't fully committed to our mother. Not that he's unwilling. He's simply unable.

It was also the day a man named Patrick Rabbitt moved his wife, Sandy, to Isle at Watercrest. Though the Rabbitts and Powes are very different families, threads of dementia weave a similar pattern.

In March of 2016, while we were in the throes of confusion and disruption with Daddy's head injury, Mom's dementia, and Tommy's and Michelle's bouts of depression, Sandy Rabbitt tripped and fell on the patio of her home in Cedar Hill, Texas. She broke her wrist, which required surgery.

Leading up to that injury, however, is a story we're all too familiar with. Patrick started picking up on Sandy's confusion with smaller, everyday things, such as road signs.

Until recently, traffic lights have been pretty straightforward—either green, yellow, or red. Then, many cities adopted the lighted arrows indicating *turn only* while simultaneously posting the solid green, yellow, or red for traffic on the straightaway.

Such subtle changes were too much for Sandy and, soon enough, Patrick took on all the driving. And then, her fall happened.

After four days in the hospital, following her surgery, Sandy was upside down.

"She couldn't walk," Patrick said. He learned the anesthesia and surgery had significantly increased the risk of dementia onset.

Several well-known studies show the risk of developing dementia nearly double within three to seven years following surgery, and of those studied, the onset is more likely to occur in women than men by almost two to one. For Sandy to go from physically functioning to unable to walk within four days was startling, but not unheard of.

Sandy underwent four weeks of rehabilitation to learn to walk again but, as we saw with our own father, a trauma reared dementia's ugly head and the battle was on.

Patrick set Sandy up with in-home care for another seven and a half weeks until he was forced to move her to Isle at Watercrest.

How do you tell a man how very lucky he is to have found Isle right from the start when he's only just beginning to process the loss of his wife?

You don't.

Knowing he and his family, and his beautiful wife, will never have to endure the horrors on the other side of memory care is a good thing while they take on the brutality of Alzheimer's. That, in of itself, is enough.

The night Sandy and I met, Isle at Watercrest was hosting its first ever art show. The manager, Patrick Peerenboom (an awesome angel placed here on Earth to care for those who cannot care for themselves), and sales coordinator, Amanda Dudziak (an awesome angel placed here on Earth to care for those who cannot care for themselves), orchestrated the event after learning Sandy was once an accomplished painter. That kind gesture turned into a fundraiser, allowing Sandy's family to show off her work while also raising money for an education scholarship where Sandy used to teach art. The showing bore beautiful results.

Art lovers who had never personally met Sandy but owned some of her work turned out and, caring not one bit that Sandy was at the height of her Alzheimer's/dementia, delighted in meeting the amazing artist.

On several occasions, it was clear that Sandy understood the event was in her honor and everyone came to see her work. When we thanked her for allowing us to see her paintings, she smiled graciously and appeared pleased. When we all laughed over some of her husband's jokes, she even joined in. How much she understood, we couldn't know, but it felt good having her sharing the experience. Standing in the reception area, surrounded by countless paintings and a good-sized crowd of friends, family, and fans of the artist, Sandy Rabbitt became very real.

I understood the sentiment as I listened to one, then another, and another speak. Before coming to Isle at Watercrest, Michelle and I told as many Marc and Colonel Powe stories as we could. We were desperate for caregivers to see our father as a man, not a patient, not a resident. And when Mom joined him, we told an equal number of Karen stories. We wanted Mom to be more than a job for them. However effective the stories may have been, or not, we always had to try. We learned Patrick had first laid eyes on Sandy when he had been but sixteen years old and she "had a really nice figure." She had been a majorette! He'd asked her out on a date, which led to two, then three, and before long, they were going steady. When his senior ring had come in, he'd worn it for exactly one day before it had gone on a chain around Sandy's neck where it had remained for the rest of high school. He'd changed colleges so he could graduate from Oklahoma State with her—she with a Bachelor of Arts in Education, he with an industrial engineering degree.

We all had a good laugh when he revealed that only after they had married in the summer of 1961 had Sandy confessed her new last name had almost been a deal breaker.

"She didn't know if she could go through life as a Mrs. Rabbitt!" Patrick said.

Sandy laughed with us on that one, too.

Her son, Steve, along with his own daughter, Sandy and Patrick's granddaughter, Rachel, were also in attendance, which was how I learned that Steve and his sister, Jenny, who died from breast cancer in December, had both been adopted.

Ann Boggs and Louise Julius, former neighbors and friends of Sandy's, shared stories about playing Bridge together and their group of friends would sneak into Sandy's studio, leaving five dollars or so as payment, any time they discovered new paintings.

"But that changed when she went to the Upstairs Gallery!" Ann said.

While the Upstairs Gallery is known to be a prestigious gallery in Arlington, Texas, Sandy's reputation as a watercolorist is known well beyond. Her showings were numerous and her ability and need to paint were insatiable.

Suddenly, Sandy was no longer a victim of Alzheimer's and dementia, she was this extraordinary woman who gave her love and talent of art to elementary school children, who not only adopted her own children but then helped Steve find his biological parents and encouraged a relationship with them. She saw shapes and shadows, colors, and details that the rest of us did not.

When Ann commented on Patrick and Sandy "always being together"—how he had driven her everywhere and how very few husbands would have gone clothing shopping with their wives as Patrick had—I wondered if Patrick loved Sandy as much as my father had once loved my mother.

Of course, I do not know Sandy, not really. I listened to stories about her, and I admired her talent, but I do not know her. Yet, I now hold a very strong feeling for her and her family. I also own one of her paintings as a reminder. But I did know the reason Patrick drove his wife around, even though I didn't mention anything to Sandy's old friends. I also recognized that Patrick was protecting Sandy in the same way Daddy had protected Mom.

How many more stories are out there just like this? How many more Powes and Rabbitts are there? No one really talks about it.

When I proposed an article featuring Sandy Rabbitt to a well-known Dallas/Fort Worth area magazine—one I have probably written more than one hundred articles for—I was saddened to have the pitch denied. Because Sandy was in the very advanced stages of the disease, and there was no happy ending to her story, the magazine declined. I quite disagreed but didn't have enough leverage to argue for the article to run.

Not celebrating extraordinary human beings because of a medical diagnosis is not only unhelpful, it is damaging.

By the year 2050, it is predicted that more than 16 million Americans will be living with this disease. And while so many don't believe this is a pressing issue or that it doesn't affect them, it does. Alzheimer's costs the United States an estimated $260 billion a year. By 2040, this disease will cost taxpayers $1.1 trillion each year. It is the sixth leading cause of death, killing more people than breast and prostate cancer victims combined. Yet, comparatively speaking, there is

no treatment and very little research.

This affects us all, but no one wants to talk about it. One reason is because it is reality and it is

scary. We want to see Sandy Rabbitt's beautiful artwork, but we don't want to see the condition

the artist is currently in. But how does this help us better understand the disease, find a treatment,

or learn proper care for those who suffer from dementia?

And it is not only the final stages of dementia that frighten but the initial stages as well.

When behaviors change, there is confusion. When there is diagnosis, there is preparation. We

need to talk about statistics, needed medications, long-term care, and caregivers. I've done

enough research at this point to know there are scores of articles and blogs dedicated to choosing

a memory-care facility, and what to look for in a caregiver, just as there are many advice

columns and support groups that ready family members for tough topics, such as memory loss,

incontinence, paranoia, new research and medicines, and unpredictable situations such as your

father suddenly stripping off all his clothing. But no one and nothing can really prepare a loved

one for the worst of it all—the in-between. The drifting paradox between worlds of dementia and

reality, where it hurts them most when they come back to us and it hurts us when they leave.

So, the stories we share with caregivers and doctors, nurses and aids, other family members, and

even each other are so crucial. They are *not* Alzheimer's patients but people *with* Alzheimer's.

Daddy *isn't* brain damaged but, rather, he *has* a damaged brain.

I was reminded of this extremely significant point, once again, by the Isle caregivers.

It cannot be emphasized enough how important it is to find quality, caring professionals, and we

understand now that the women at the previous facilities were unhappy in their work. Truly,

these professionals are not paid enough for everything they do! Our police officers, educators, and care professionals should be making quadruple the money, and our pro athletes and celebs,

who are playing games, need to be scaled *way* down.

I digress. Again.

The professionals who hate their jobs then take it out on their elderly charges while the staff at

Isle at Watercrest restore dignity. They also share stories.

One day, sitting in the dining area with my father, my mother and sister walked in after hanging

together while I tried to talk to Daddy.

Mom walked up and gave Daddy several kisses on his face, and Thelma cooed.

"Sometimes Karen gets jealous when we take care of Marc, but we are all so jealous of Karen!

Oh, I want that! Why can't I have that?" Thelma laughed as she explained how often Mom and

Daddy cuddle, how many times Daddy picks up her hands to kiss each and every finger, how

they sit together for hours without speaking but are just content in each other's company. "We

are so jealous of Ms. Karen."

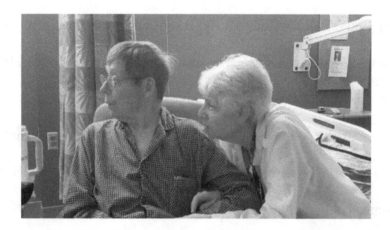

This picture, taken by Michelle, is a classic Marc & Karen shot—hip-to-hip—riveted by a game. They loved baseball, soccer, and the Olympics.

Chapter Fourteen

FACEBOOK: *April 2017*

> *NOT advisable: While staying in a locked memory-care facility, after you've been up all night with your dad and you're super tired and he finally goes to bed, DO NOT sprawl out on the floor so that the night nurse comes in…in the dark…and sees the silhouette of a body on the ground.*
> *Apparently, this is upsetting to the staff!*
> *#NightNurseCalling911 #SorryNightNurse*

What is dementia anyway?

For those moments when they are coherent, Mom more so than Daddy, it is bittersweet. When they are with us, it is so wonderful and amazing, which only makes the confusion and faraway looks that much more painful. The worst, however, is when they recognize their own inability to grasp some thought that is almost within reach. The look of confusion then frustration, the dropped shoulders, stammering for words, and then the heavy sigh and final resignation are so hard to endure. That's when I typically become very silly, hoping to distract.

As I type these very words, I am sitting in their room, on a Sunday evening, with plans to spend the night. While we rode high on the roller coaster, high on the idea that Daddy was getting better, talking once more, and Mom was finally socially interacting, the fun is coming to an end. Mom's Alzheimer's is a restless beast that seeks only to make everyone miserable.

For the first time in my life, I watched my mother scream. And at our beloved Maria, no less. Maria is another earthbound angel my parents adore—when they remember to.

For whatever reasons, Mom began refusing showers about three weeks prior. Simple prodding was no longer enough, so when I came for a regular visit, Maria suggested maybe I could bribe Mom into taking a shower.

At first, our suggestions were diplomatic. "Everyone needs a shower!"

"You want to smell nice for Daddy, right?"

But this only irritated her. "I just *had* a shower!" On that, you could not convince her otherwise.

So, we moved to a new phase of delicate suggestion. "Um, well, you…ah, well, Mom…you

don't, uh, well…you don't smell all that good.

Stand back. She's whirling! She's whirling!

Of late, we've been reduced to the kind of bribes and trickery used on our children. "If you take

a shower, we can have some pizza."

"If you take a shower, we can go out."

"If you take a shower, we'll…"

On this particular day, she mentioned a hamburger, and Maria and I pounced. "Sure! Here, why

don't you take a shower, and then I'll take you out for a burger."

Maria and I secretly shot hand signals back and forth, and so confident we had this in the bag, I

slipped out to find Daddy, waited about ten minutes, and then headed back to the room. *We will*

go out, get her a burger an—

Mom stood, stark naked, in the middle of her room, screaming at Maria.

I rushed forward, shocked. "What? What happened?"

Maria said nothing. She looked uncharacteristically flustered.

What I did not yet know was that Mom had hit Maria. Repeat: Mom hit Maria.

To Maria's credit, she never said a word. She only told me that Mom was very upset with her

and asked if, perhaps, I could help dress her.

Yes. Of course. I turned to Mom still confident I could save the day. I handed Mom her bra.

"Let's get dressed."

She ripped the bra from my hands and threw it with impressive velocity on the floor. "That is *not*

my bra."

Okay. "Let's get you dressed."

I tried again, but she came very close to my face and began yelling at me.

"Why would you allow that to happen? I have never been so humiliated in all my life!" She

screamed at me for not helping, for not stopping Maria.

"I asked Maria to bathe you, Mom. I'm sorry. But you need—"

"Why would you do that?"

Expounding upon the reasons she needed a shower—that she did not smell good and hygiene

was an issue, that she would feel better once she was clean—were not only pointless statements,

they were agitators.

Instead, I said, "Let's get dressed and go out for burgers."

"I have no clothes!"

"You have a closet full of—"

"I HAVE NO CLOTHES!"

"Ah, but you do."

She eyed me with suspicion.

"I went by the store on my way up here and got you some new clothes."

She eased toward the closet, peered inside, and instantly recognized the everything hanging

inside. "Those are *my* clothes," she snapped.

I went for a new tact—relief. "Oh, *yeah.* Nice. Good eye, Mom, good eye! Here. You pick out

what to wear. You always look so cute. Everyone always talks about how cute you look."

Boy, she really thought about that one. She sighed heavily, leaned into to the closet, and pointed

at a crewneck pinstriped sweater. "That one."

"Again, excellent eye!" And I spent the rest of the afternoon trying to maintain that level of enthusiasm as she told me she had never in her life eaten a chicken sandwich (*Well, by golly! Let's go get you a chicken sandwich!*), she had never been in my car before (*Well, by golly, let's drive around, and I'll show you how the stereo and phone system work!*), and Michelle never comes to visit her (*Well, she's always been a brat!* [Hahahaha!])

Later, however, she shared a very detailed story on the name *Lily* and its history within our family.

No matter how much I tried to preserve and savor the moment, the reality was we were in a mad game of peek-a-boo. I was shown brief moments of clarity then we were back to great declarations of nonsensical things.

Just as Alzheimer's has Mom madly pulling things from her closet at 3 am or hiding everything, claiming her husband is having an affair, or denying ever doing or seeing or eating or wearing things she has, Daddy's confusion makes him aggressive.

We have great theories and hypotheses, Michelle and I. We believe Mom's 2 and 3 am closet raids, with its side of complementary bright light, cause agitation for our father. We suspect the caregivers on the night shift are so focused on their jobs, such as changing our father's diaper, that, in the moment, they come at him too quickly and too aggressively. We also believe his medication may not be right. The reality is, however, while all of the above may be true, we're also losing our father to dementia and brain damage.

On this particular night in a locked-in facility, though, Daddy is not only quiet but he is very sweet. But he has not been so sweet to others, hence my reason for being here.

Between the hours of 10 pm, Friday evening, and 5 am, Saturday morning, for whatever reason, he walked the hallways, rattling doors and trying to escape. He had physical altercations that later confused and upset him, greatly concerned the staff, and devastated us. It also triggered the facility to institute a new policy—all doors of each resident are locked every night to keep him from getting in to other people's rooms.

Still, it wasn't enough, and Isle asked that we take our father to a psychiatric hospital for evaluation.

On a Sunday morning, Michelle and I packed enough clothing for five days, collected his various medications, and wrestled him into my car during a torrential downpour.

At the hospital, we filled out paperwork and entertained/distracted our father until, at last, we were called.

The intake nurse asked just three questions: What is your name? Do you know where you are? Do you know why you are here?

Even as she asked, Michelle and I looked at each other.

Was she kidding? Why did I just fill out lines and lines of paperwork describing his inability to speak, answer appropriately, and understand where he was or what he was doing from one minute to the next?

She straightened again. "We can't admit him. He can't speak for himself."

Well, duh. That's why we're here.

The only reason we had even made the difficult trip was because Isle at Watercrest had asked us to. We wanted to show them good faith. We wanted them to see we're more than willing to work with them, possibly discover what was wrong with our father and, if possible, save him.

What no one had mentioned up until this point was that we could not admit a person to a psychiatric hospital unless I had guardianship. I had an executive Power of Attorney but not guardianship.

Hear me now, folks, these are *not* the same thing. They do not grant the same authorities.

Our entire drive back to Isle, Michelle and I fretted that Daddy would not be welcomed.

What if this was all a ruse to just get him out?

We panicked and called Isle to let them know we were returning with two thoughts drumming through our brains: *We can't move Mom again. She is already losing it and to disorient her yet again would be cruel beyond measure.* But the more pressing concern was if we had to move Daddy again, where we would go. *Who would take him?*

As we rolled up, however, Wendy from Human Resources, an always smiling, sweet, pretty woman who got into memory care because of her own family, welcomed us.

I wanted to cry. I would have but those ducts went dry about eight months ago.

There was, however, a condition—we had to sit with our father during night hours.

Memories flooded back. Our hell was about to start all over again, but that sliver of hope dangled before us, like bait, so we set about figuring it out. With Robb traveling the upcoming week, I decided to take Sunday night and Michelle agreed to Monday.

Just before Michelle left, she got the honor of being kicked in the stomach by her father. Literally.

To his credit, it was mostly a warning shot. Again, he needed to have his diaper changed but being modest and fearful of being naked, he would not allow his pants to be removed under any circumstances.

While Michelle was attempting to help a caregiver, Daddy looked right at her and said, "Michelle! You need to do better."

Whoa.

Another guest of the Isle is a known skipper. She skips, or more specifically, hops, down the halls. When it comes time for her to be showered and/or changed, however, she bolts. Upon leaving the shower, still slick from the water and naked as a jaybird, she can sometimes be hard to catch and will race of her room and tear down the hallway.

I'm sorry to say this, but…it's hilarious, and I desperately wish Daddy would take up streaking, not punching and kicking.

Around 1 am that morning, one of the night-shift caregivers came in, and I saw his agitation play out. Daddy's diaper was full. I could smell the urine from my seat next to him, in our matching recliners. No doubt, he had to be changed.

But as the woman came in, her voice louder than warranted, Daddy went on instant alert. She was very pleasant but headed straight for him.

Daddy quickly stood and began easing behind the chair, not making eye contact.

I wanted to say, *He's okay. Leave him alone.* But the reality was he *needed* to be changed. So, I helpfully fussed as I silently prayed he would be agreeable.

He was not.

When a second caregiver came in, I watched his spine stiffen and his jaw set.

Shit. "Daddy, it's okay. You need to be changed." My comments were useless.

He was in complete defense mode, ready to fight, to save himself from the demons only he imagined before him.

Why can't he understand what angels they are?

They were an incredible tag team. In less than eight minutes, they had him changed and back in dry diapers, pajama bottoms on, all while ducking and dodging possible blows.

As they left, Christeen said, "He's really mad."

When I was little, and even not so little, I entertained my parents as they nestled in bed with their books. I danced back and forth past the doorway of their room, disappearing and then re-appearing, with an imaginary cane and top hat, tap dancing as I went. The tap dance turned into a tango then a waltz, the mashed-potato, and the pony. I ended each show with my own rendition of a strung-out rock star's air-guitar solo until they were laughing so hard, and one of them would finally yell, "Go to bed!"

On this night, securely locked inside Isle at Watercrest, I tried dancing down memory lane once again. While Mom and Daddy sat on their recliners, I performed Swan Lake, the robot, a one-woman tango, and finished with a tap dance that would have made Gene Kelly proud. I got both parents rolling with laughter.

It felt amazing. Also, a little exhausting because no one ever told me to go to bed.

Instead, Mom gave in and went to bed, leaving Daddy and I to watch Law & Order (Oh, the irony) until after three in the morning.

When he finally stood, I asked if he wanted to go to bed.

"Mm-hm."

Good enough for me.

But as we walked into their bedroom, our nemesis, Alzheimer's, was raring to go and we found Mom, dressed and making her bed.

I let her know Daddy was going to bed.

"Oh, no he's not. I just made this bed!"

"Mom, it's three in the morning. Everyone is sleeping."

She was indignant. "Well, not in here, they aren't!"

Too tired to tap dance any longer, I went for the compromise instead. "Let Daddy sleep here, and you can sit with me. I have a secret to tell you about Daddy."

In the weeks following, as Michelle and I quickly burned out, we spent nearly five thousand more dollars a month for private sitter care.

Our quandary was real. We desperately tried to find a new, better, different diagnosis for our father to alleviate his aggression, but Mom was not endearing herself to anyone. Her Alzheimer's was enveloping her. She was more often mean than nice, confused than clear, and paranoid than certain.

While the day shift adored my father, the night shift did not.

One night, Daddy kept pointing out a blank wall. It was bare. Nothing on it. But something about the wall bothered him so greatly that he and I began our dance. I ran my hands over it, show him there was nothing there, and we shrugged at each other until, a minute later, he indicated some problem with the wall again.

Is this simply brain damage, or is it also sundowners? Does his kind of brain damage and hydrocephalus cause him to see things?

Yet another time, he continued insistently pointing out something on the floor.

I saw nothing but floor.

It agitated him so greatly, however, so I walked back and forth, hopping on the very spot he'd pointed to, as he watched with intense interest. Classic Alzheimer's.

Once again, Michelle and I devised a plan: *Operation Diagnosis.*

Because Daddy's medical history is so complicated, we are not only at constant war with the medical teams of Isle, Dr. Moody, and the VA, as well as the medical team of the VA's primary caregiver, we are also at odds with private home-health agencies and different caregivers. Everyone has a different opinion why Daddy is behaving as he is.

Ever his knight, Michelle could not let go of the idea that the hydrocephalus was adding pressure to an already bruised brain. Her theory involved having a procedure to release the water on his brain. She was certain he would improve even more. Maybe releasing pressure would help him behaviorally. Maybe the procedure would increase stability, return his speech, and revitalize cognition. Maybe we could get him back. Maybe it wasn't too late. We'd accepted Mom's diagnosis of Alzheimer's, but Daddy…his was more complicated, more specialized, more hopeful.

So, once again, I strapped on my Super Woman cape and announced, "I'm going in!" My plan? Calling the VA and boldly securing a neurologist appointment for my father. "We are going to get to the bottom of this once and for all."

I woke early, eager and optimistic. First, call the pharmacy at Veterans Affairs in hopes of learning exactly what medications my dad was taking, who had prescribed what and when, and then, armed with the most up-to-date information, double back ready to take on the Neurology department.

The VA pharmacy refused to recognize me as Power of Attorney.

But I was ready. I'd had this exact fight five times during the prior months. I sent a twenty-page Power of Attorney document—notarized *and* certified with the state of Texas and identified by not one but two different lawyers as "one of the most detailed and thorough POAs I've ever seen"—to the officers of Veterans Affairs in Wisconsin, Minnesota, and Washington D.C. I also hand delivered a copy to the Green Team of the Dallas VA and gave a copy to the head of the neurology department and the physician's assistant.

But, alas…apparently, this was not enough.

Never mind that the Silver Team, the Green Team, the neurology departments, along with the hearing (aids) and eye team of the VA all recognized me, and never mind that my father was physically and mentally incapable of explaining who he was and what he needed. I was told he had to do just that.

I went back to the Silver Team, who referred me to the Release of Information Department.

Ah, yes, my friends, the Release of Information.

At ROI, I was told she was not able to release information to anyone except…the Power of Attorney.

Um. "But…I *am* the POA."

She said she needed authorized documentation.

"But you have it!"

I was sent to the Department of Eligibility—where it was determined that I was, indeed, eligible to discuss my father's medical issues—then transferred back to Release of Information for yet another standoff.

After surviving what felt like the verbal equivalent of fifteen rounds with Rhonda Rousey, I shared this tidbit. "I'm tweeting this entire conversation…"

In the course of this past year, I have learned Twitter is my friend. While I don't stay up late at night, tweeting out hateful words against those who oppose my way of thinking, *al la* some of our fearful leaders, I do question ethics. And with all we've been through with Mom and Daddy, after weeks of trying to settle something privately, I have tweeted companies, organizations, politicians, and private groups who can't seem to keep their sticky fingers out of my father's wallet. The response is amazing. Privately, they don't care. Make it public, however, and the apologies rain down like a much-needed storm on a hot summer day—complete with rainbows and fluffy clouds.

"I'm tweeting this entire conversation live, because no one will believe what is going on…"

I was directed back to the pharmacy and told, "You need to go to Release of Information."

I did not yell. I did not curse. I didn't even tweet. I simply said, "Okay, just listen, for one second. Don't look at your screen or anyone around you. Just hear my words and pretend like I'm a friend of yours."

She became quiet, and I went through the list of departments I'd been, who had been given what, and exactly what the deal was.

I have to give her this—she did seem to care.

She gave me the name of the Chief of Pharmacy and apologized, as this truly was the best she could do.

"I'll take it and thanks."

Somehow, I ended up at the VA in Topeka, Kansas, with an exceptionally rude woman who not only refused to hear me out but also interrupted me several times just to say, "Listen to me!" She was so convinced I wasn't listening that she never seemed to hear me repeatedly say I had already spoken to Release of Information and the Department of Inquiry and the Patient's Advocacy Department and the pharmacy multiple times. She was on a roll.

I shut up and let her direct me to all the places I had already visited multiple times until she, at long last, ended by telling me I needed to go to Eligibility.

I tried a new tactic. "I can't."

"Why?"

"I've already been to all those places. I've spent the last hour and twenty minutes on the phone, going through this with each department, and I want to cry because all I want is for my dad—a man who served his country faithfully and selflessly for more than three decades—to be cared for." I explained that my POA was a great one, but only half the VA seemed capable of recognizing it, and if I went back to Eligibility, they *would* recognize me, but as soon as I went to Release of Information, they would not…and thus, a new cycle was destined to begin all over again. "Could you call Eligibility on my behalf and have *them* tell you I'm really the real deal?"

"Please hold." When she returned, she seemed very pleased to inform me that I was real.

After nearly an hour and a half on the phone, I got the answer to the only question I had—*Yes, we can send your father's medical file and medications to the neurology department.*

A month and many more similarly aggravating conversations later, a VA appointment was set for Daddy to get updated on his medical status, possible evaluation on neurological and behavioral issues, and medications.

Despite our frustrations, we love the VA. Daddy feels, pardon the pun-ny expression, *at ease* at the VA. When we take Daddy to an appointment, any appointment, we are immensely aware of how the day might go. It could be easy, or it might turn into a genuine WWF throw down. At the VA, we don't worry quite as much since there is no shortage of help. More importantly, he is among his people—enlisted and officer, male and female, young and old. Marc Powe loves the soldier. We do, too.

On the day of his appointment, however, we were not prepared for an overnight stay. But with respect to the opinion of the physician's assistant, Wanda Novak, we agreed. But we had some conditions.

"He's going to need his own private room and a full-time sitter," Michelle instructed as I nodded enthusiastically.

Oh, but even after all we have been through and all that we know, there are disbelievers. *How bad could the Colonel be? He looks so sweet and polite.*

When we got to the sixth floor and discovered Daddy was sharing a room with another patient and there was no sitter, Michelle and I exchanged glances. One should never doubt the wisdom of my sister when it came to the Colonel's medical care.

"He can't share a room."

I'm sure, in her mind, the polite nurse was merely advising us about room availability and their standards and guidelines for watching him and—

But this is how it really went down:

> Nurse: Blah, blah, blah…
>
> Daddy: [pulls back curtain and peers intently at the patient sleeping on the other side]
>
> Nurse: …blah, blah, blah, blah…
>
> Daddy: [moves toward machine connected to other patient and promptly turns it off]
>
> Nurse: …blah, blah, bla—[looks a little alarmed]
>
> Michelle: [surprisingly unruffled by our father's assault on other patient's machine, turns it back on]
>
> Daddy: [turns machine off again and moves in for closer inspection of now-waking other patient]
>
> Michelle: [flips machine back on] Yeah, we're really going to need another room.
>
> Nurse: …
>
> Daddy: [finds remote to something and starts jabbing buttons]

Michelle: [retrieves remote from Daddy's hands] He's not going to stop. Not ever.

Wife of other patient: [looks alarmed]

Other patient: [now wide awake and alarmed]

Daddy: [Not at all alarmed but determined to further inspect other patient's medical condition]

Michelle: [redirects Daddy] And we're going to need a sitter because Alex and I have to leave soon.

Note: This is a fantastic strategy Michelle and I have learned throughout the course of this journey—saying we are about to leave Marc Powe in *your* hands, and then standing back and watching the looks ranging from mild terror to outright horror cross a person's face when they realize they are about to be left alone with Colonel Marc Powe – the man, the myth, the memory-care legend.

Nurse: [anticipated look of mild terror crosses her face]

Daddy: [standing over other patient]

Other patient: [look of terror crosses over the MILD bridge and rapidly steps onto the VERGE OF HYSTERIA shoreline]

Daddy: [says something inaudible to terrified other patient]

Michelle: And once he takes an interest in something…

Daddy: [flips machine off]

Michelle: [flips machine back on]

Daddy: [flips machine off again]

Wife of other patient: [jaw drops. It's clear she wants to speak but isn't sure what to say.]

> Michelle: [gestures toward open-mouthed wife of other patient] This isn't fair to them
>
> either.
>
> Daddy: [flips machine off again]

Daddy got a private room and a sitter, a Navy corpsman named Joshua.

Clearly, Joshua had received prior warning about Colonel Powe. By the time he got to our room,

he appeared ready to block doors and redirect.

We explained Daddy would be staying overnight for observation, lab work, and a full assessment

with the neurology team.

We had a lot of questions in need of answers. Was this because of the head trauma? The

hydrocephalus? Both? Or were those white spots on the brain scan we had heard about, but never

seen, been indicators of Parkinson's? How much of this was possibly due to the radiation Soviets

blasted into the American Embassy? We knew a ventricle vein in the brain was enlarged and that

there seemed to be some atrophy, but was it from the dementia? The head trauma? Something

else?

As we pondered our never-ending list of growing questions, Daddy pondered a new escape route

by opening the window.

Michelle was updating Joshua on Daddy's affectations—tells that he's readying himself for

another escape—when she looked up to see our father breaking into the wall-mounted

evacuation kit that inflates a giant yellow slide.

Together, they wrestled Daddy away from the encased rubber slide, and the young Navy

corpsman planted his body squarely in front of the door so Daddy couldn't escape.

Our father may have wandered aimlessly and endlessly through the memory care, but the VA

hospital was a different ballgame altogether. He was supposed to remain in his own room.

He, however, did not see it that way. Colonel Marc Powe shuffled toward the door for his first standoff with Joshua and gestured for the young man to move.

Joshua didn't give an inch.

Daddy gestured again.

"No can do, sir."

Another gesture.

"No, sir."

"Navy, move over there!"

Joshua and Michelle burst into laughter at Daddy's clear order. Daddy didn't know the guy's name, but by golly, he knew he was Navy!

During the next twenty-four hours, the night nurse—our personal welcome wagon upon arrival and witness to Daddy spending time in semi-private rooms—requested a different gig, wanting no part of our father again, and the second nurse had to be replaced once she saw wrestling *was* actually part of her job description that night.

Joshua, however, came back to us the following day, as did the neurology team—with news that was stunning, unsettling, greatly needed, and liberating.

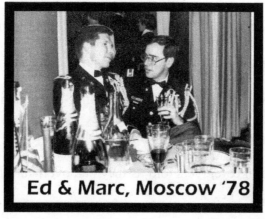

Ed & Marc, Moscow '78

Another rare picture of the then Lt. Col Powe with one of his best friends, Col. Ed Baisden, stationed in Moscow, Russia

Chapter Fifteen

FACEBOOK: *July 2017*

> *That moment when your mother is extremely agitated, claiming she no longer has any underwear or other unmentionables, but you know she does because you just bought some and you are prepared to say as much when you look over and see your father trying to put **her** underwear over **his** shoe.*
> *Do you say, "No, Daddy! That's not a sock. That's mom's underwear!"*
> *Or do you say, "Mom, look out the window! It's Judy Garland, from the Wizard of Oz...and Toto too!"*

While Daddy was, at long last, receiving a full assessment from a neurology team, Mom was pacing the halls of Isle at Watercrest, husbandless and afraid. Two words which had been recurring topics for many months.

When they had still been living at the other place—the bad place—Mom had insisted Daddy was asking for a divorce but we hadn't believed her.

Who would? First of all, no man has ever loved his wife more than Marc Powe loves Karen, and second, he couldn't talk.

But she had been adamant, and we had pooh-poohed her. We'd told her she misunderstood, that he hadn't meant it...he hadn't known what he was saying.

But at Isle, once Daddy settled in and began trusting people, he also began speaking again.

That was when Londa approached me. "Your dad asked me to marry him."

I replied just as any person in my position would. "I'm not calling you 'Mom'."

When I told Michelle, however, she was horrified. Her knee-jerk reaction was, "Oh, my God. She's been telling us he was saying that but we didn't believe her."

To make matters worse, several caregivers told us they had overheard Daddy vocalizing the word *divorce* to Mom.

While Michelle empathized with Mom, I wondered about Daddy. If there was any credence to the stories, how long had those feelings been festering?

There was no denying, throughout the years, she mistreated him. Now, with a head injury and free of any obligations to anyone or anything, he was a free man.

He's always enjoyed wandering, doing his own thing. He likes being alone. In fact, Daddy's favorite thing is getting up early, grabbing a cup of coffee, and simply sitting. Sometimes he writes (nonsensical things) or reads the newspaper. Other times, he appears content just watching the world go by.

I am my father's daughter. I so understand that. I love getting up super early, while the world is still mostly asleep and quiet. It is a time when no one wants or needs anything from you.

In the wee hours, Daddy was always a free man.

Whatever he is doing, however, Mom can't stand it. She tugs, pulls, pushes, and pesters him. He is her new Colby, the dog she could never ever leave alone. When he wanders at 2 am, she tries to pull him back into the room. When he moves furniture, she engages in what must be (for him) an infuriating game of tug-of-couch, though it's highly amusing to the rest of us. And when he just wants peace, she hovers. Always, she hovers. So, yeah. He wants a divorce.

Ever so briefly, we discussed the idea of separating them. Perhaps if they were living in separate quarters, they could both be happier.

It is my intention with this book to not only highlight the toll this disease has on entire families and communities but also discuss the value of care giving. By and large, these are professionals who are grossly underpaid and undervalued. The result is too many unqualified and/or ill-equipped people (mostly women) get into this field believing it to be a relatively easy gig. The training they receive is inadequate. Memory care is *not* just about changing diapers, pushing people around in wheelchairs, and staying on a strict feeding schedule. It is about remembering that these seemingly mindless people are, in fact, people. They have amazing stories, families, children, and grandchildren. They did cool things. And, however "out of it" they may appear to be, there are often times of coherency in which they still know and understand fear and love, humor and worry. They get confused and scared. They wish they were home and have cravings for chocolate or something hot. They want, just for one damned second, to have a choice in what they do, eat, wear, or where they walk. Yet they regularly have some twenty-seven-year-old mother (oftentimes single), who is worn out and not being paid enough to have a wrestling match over a sock or a stapler or a fork, handling them—literally and figuratively —with every move they make, and they get pissed. These nurses/aids/sitters/caregivers only see a brain diseased, confused elderly person who won't even remember this particular battle twenty minutes from now, and so they speak their mind, saying things that are too harsh or unkind. Worse, they don't talk at all because…what's the point? This senile old bat won't remember anyway, right?

I wish it was a federal law that all people in the memory-care business were required to pass college coursework when working with a person with dementia, not to be confused with a person with Alzheimer's, not to be confused with working with a person with head trauma or Parkinson's or bipolar or vascular disorders or multiple sclerosis…

I wish there was a required number of hours a caregiver had to complete in compassion and communication.

I also wish I had running video footage of my parents between the hours of 10 pm and 6 am. I could speed it up so it looked like they were moving super-fast, and I would post it on YouTube and make millions.

But I digress.

The women who care for our parents now are incredible. One after another states it in the simplest terms. "You have to understand dementia." They explain it is the dementia that makes their residents nice one minute and mean the next. It is dementia that brings about the confusion, frustration, fear, and anxiety, and when one of the more unpleasant characteristics rears its ugly head, the staff doesn't think Mom or Sylvia or Trent or Daddy are horrible, rotten people. They know it is the disease.

This is so important.

With proper training, both sides win. The patient and the family can both breathe easier knowing the caregiver isn't taking bad behaviors personally. We are so grateful for this. Our loved ones are treated with understanding, patience, and love rather than frustration, anger, and animosity. The caregiver wins as well. When he or she truly understands the disease, they can compartmentalize Karen Powe, the person, from Karen Powe, the victim. Karen Powe, the person, is a kind and giving woman. Karen Powe, the victim, is exhausting and becoming increasingly frightened and needy.

If our parents were separated, Mom could stop obsessing over Daddy and Daddy could finally be at peace.

It would be so easy for the staff to say, "Yes! Please, dear Lord in Heaven, separate them! Send your mother away!"

They didn't. Not one person said yes to the idea of separating them to the point that Mom and Daddy could never see each other again. Rather, the debate was *do we keep them in the same room but separate beds?* Or *do we put them in separate bedrooms and they can see each other during the day?*

We had more discussions with more caregivers, doctors, counselors, and other Alzheimer/dementia survivors on the subject of physically separating our parents than I could possibly recount. Daddy is next on the waiting list for his own private room but all the caregivers were evenly divided on the subject.

Ultimately, we decided to make a change, and for the first time in more than fifty years, they were sleeping in separate beds.

Briefly, during the days when Mom was still coherent as much as 40 percent of the time, she said she wanted the divorce too. She was embarrassed by Daddy's constant movement, late-night walkabouts, and his new need to strip his pants before taking to the halls. Sometimes she held those feelings for as much as a day.

And so, began *Operation Divorce*.

Michelle began planting the idea that Mom didn't need Daddy, that she was her own woman, while I reinforced our mission objective by giving Mom a semblance of control.

"Say the word," I told her, "and I'll put all the money in your account only."

We even had a friend, a retired lawyer, agree to draw up mock divorce papers Mom could sign and be free.

While we were still entertaining the idea of physically separating our parents' rooms, one deterrent kept popping up—Karen would find her husband, no matter what. We knew this was true.

One particular day, Mom, Daddy, and I were outside on the patio while Daddy busily and happily rearranged all the patio furniture.

Mom ramped up, telling me I had to stop him. He was going to make "the people" mad. Always, his activity, no matter what it was, was a trigger for Mom. She became frantic, first pulling on me. "Alex! Alex! He's [fill in the blank]. Alex, stop him before [fill in the blank]."

This escalated to outer-realm things.

> Mom: He's going to wake the children!
>
> Alex: What children?
>
> Mom: The children! They live here, too.
>
> Alex: Oh, no, Mom. Maybe some come to visit, but there aren't any children who live here.
>
> Mom: I think I know what I've seen, and there are children who live here.
>
> Alex: [knowing I can't argue with her, tries logic] Well, it's almost noon. They're all awake.
>
> Mom: But they are trying to sleep now. Your father kept them awake all night!

Unable to settle her down, I suggested she and I go get a Coke. She usually loved that. On this day, however, she wasn't so sure, but I pulled out every trick I had and finally got her to leave Daddy to his re-arranging.

By the time we got to the other side of the building, Mom caught a glimpse of Daddy through the double doors, and she became frantic. She charged the door and began wildly—and I mean *wildly*—tugging the handles.

When the doors wouldn't open (there was a large sign posted: *These Doors Do Not Open*), she banged her little fists on the glass so hard they rattled and I feared she would break them and seriously hurt herself.

"Mom. Mom! That's glass. You're going to break it!"

"You're damned right I am!" she said as she began kicking the door.

I had to physically remove her, and that was when she turned on me. It was stunning really.

I'd heard stories about my mother turning feral but it had been hard to imagine. I'd never disbelieved what I had been told. I just hadn't been able to picture it.

Remarkably, the caregivers always said the same thing. "It's okay. They don't mean it. It's not them."

Never were truer words spoken.

This isn't them. This is *not* them. This is not who they are. *Sonofabitch, but I hate Alzheimer's and dementia.*

To get a better idea of what exactly we were dealing with, when Michelle and I were asked to take a dementia tour, we agreed.

The Virtual Dementia Tour was created by geriatric specialist, P. K. Beville, CEO of Second Wind Dreams, in an attempt to provide caregivers and family members with a greater sense of how those with Alzheimer's and dementia see their world. To date, more than five hundred *thousand* people have taken the tour, and those numbers are steadily increasing as this tour is now provided in many nursing and health-care programs.

First, we were given inserts to put in our shoes, which made walking painful.

Turns out peripheral neuropathy—damage to peripheral nerves—is connected to dementia and Alzheimer's. It can cause numbness and pain, usually in the hands and feet.

Even as Amanda, our tour guide for the day, saw my expression change, she nodded. "It's why so many of our residents take off their shoes, walking around in just socks or barefoot."

It is a constant battle for the caregivers who try their absolute best to keep residents' feet covered and safe. A good many are always kicking off their shoes.

I got it now.

We were also given gloves with popcorn kernels inserted into the inner gloves to act as irritants. It was distracting and uncomfortable. But when larger gloves were placed over the others, it also became cumbersome and made finger and hand coordination difficult.

Next, we were given earplugs to impair hearing and eyewear resembling goggles. The lenses were designed to mimic the way a person with Alzheimer's and dementia saw the world.

We were led to a dimly lit room and given five tasks to complete. My tasks were clearing the table, finding a tie and putting it around my neck, drawing a picture of my family, folding/rolling up six pairs of socks, and finding then working a belt through the loops of a pair of pants.

Once inside, there was no talking and Amanda was not able to assist in any way. To top things off, some kind of radio or recorder playing sounds of static, a siren, slamming doors, a phone ringing, people talking, and something that sounded a lot like gunshots.

Right away, I found the closet and located a tie, a belt, and a pair of pants. Half my work—completed.

I cleared the table easily enough and figured out where the desk was then found a pen and some stationary to draw my picture. My feet, however...

I was also starting to sweat, and it was nearly impossible to hold the pen in my gloved hand, but I managed.

Tie. Check.

Belt in pants. Check.

Table. Check.

Drawing. Check.

What was the other thing?

Gunshot.

My feet are killing me!

Static.

Sirens.

And then, another gun shot. *I think that was a gunshot.*

People talking. *So many people talking, but what are they saying?*

Tie. Belt. Table. Drawing.

"What was that other thing?" I asked out loud. *You're not supposed to talk.*

Nothing.

I tilted my head back and forth, trying to peek past the lenses of my Mr. Magoo goggles.

Another gunshot.

Seriously, did they crank the heat in here? It's boiling. I paced around a bit, thought I saw some kind of list but was unable to read it clearly enough, and so I perched my enormous oversized-gloved hands on my hips. "Well, I give up."

What I didn't realize was that I was being scored on ability, memory, levels of frustration and/or anger, and cooperation. I was marked *frustrated* quite a few times.

Okay! I'm blind, partially deaf, someone keeps firing a gun, it's nine hundred degrees in here, and my feet are killing me! But I never cursed. At least, not so anyone heard. And aside from my inability to recall that fifth item, I performed my other tasks fairly quickly, which was better than anyone knew because, for some reason, I'd gotten it into my head that I had six tasks to perform. I wasn't supposed to, but I cheated and told Michelle what to expect so she would fare better than I had. Team Powe, all the way! *Operation Powe!*

But she cussed, talked to Amanda, then got turned around and, in a surprising move, started shadowing the other person in her test.

Oh, the irony.

Mom shadows. She walks so close behind us if we stop short, she bangs into us.

What wasn't surprising was how we both reacted afterward. We learned it is very common for participants to quit halfway through the tour, as they become overwhelmed with grief or sadness or guilt. Participants' most common recorded responses are, "I felt isolated," "I wanted someone to show me what to do," "I was frightened," "I couldn't focus on what I was supposed to do," "The sounds in my head made it impossible for me to pay attention," and "I gave up." Many family members finish the tour, however successfully or not, saying, "I had no idea that was how it felt."

I never felt isolated or scared because I knew what I was doing was just a drill, an exercise. I was mostly annoyed by the sounds and not remembering what the fifth and sixth tasks were.

Of the two of us, I am the researcher. Michelle is the mother of guilt.

I had clinical questions. *Who designed the study and why? How did they figure how bad to make the vision or hearing? How do we know their feet hurt this much? And how do we know this is how clumsy they feel?* But the bigger question—*what was that sound that sounded like a gunshot?* Answer: books being dropped.

Michelle, however, was not so analytical. She felt awful for being irritated when Mom dropped things. She felt guilty we had dismissed Mom's rising paranoia about gunshots. She was distressed by the realization that Mom's world was so dark, confusing, and chaotic. How many hours upon hours had we spent with Mom, assuming the brightly lit, yet tranquil, setting we were in was pleasant only to discover Mom's world was completely the opposite?

But didn't we already know that? I mean…how many times has Mom jumped at a noise, or become alarmed by a sudden movement, even gasped when someone handed someone else a napkin? It also explained why Mom couldn't handle sudden movements. Why she felt an insatiable need to follow then monitor every move Daddy makes. As he moves about, so do imaginary hordes of children, packs of dogs, and people with guns. She's obsessed with the idea that people are going to kill her, the existence of a basement where the guns are kept, and Daddy having secret and not-so-secret lovers. To tell her otherwise was to disrespect her, which is yet another agitator.

And she wasn't the only one.

Joan saw a dead woman in her room. She lived next to Mom and Daddy and, on any given day, could be found sobbing in the hallway and gesturing vaguely toward her room. She mumbled/cried so incoherently I regularly needed a translation to know what Joan was saying. It's still unclear if this was a dead woman Joan knew or a stranger, but it is real and horrible and frightening for, so we each took turns gently consoling and leading her away every time we saw her.

Joan is a gentle soul, tormented by the disease and, perhaps, the past, and is almost always appreciative of the reassurances.

One day, however, when I launched into my normal routine with her, first petting her arm then taking her hand and suggesting we go into the dining hall where everyone else was—"Yes, yes, I know. It is so sad," and "I'll take care of it."

She snapped at me. "Take care of it?" Joan's voice was no longer feeble and pathetic but strong and angry. "What do you mean, 'take care of it'?"

I was kind of surprised, almost embarrassed, being caught pooh-poohing her emotions and/or

what she believed to be real. "Um, I-I'm, uh, I'm gonna call the morgue?"

She just stared at me.

We, families of those who have dementia or Alzheimer's, become masters at deflecting,

redirecting, and just playing along. You have to.

Many more of us learn to find the humor. Again, you have to, or it will swallow you whole.

Mom's mental capacity is diminishing so rapidly that it's unsettling. We can't quite get our

footing. Each time we feel like we've got control, she hits a new low. She has become

increasingly unfriendly. Convinced she's being poisoned, she slaps medicine out of nurses'

hands. She refuses to eat and begs, actually pleads, with me and Michelle not to make eye

contact with other residents and caregivers, as they are all "horrid" and "cannot be trusted." It is

embarrassing and inexplicable.

While we were at the VA, however, we could only hope Mom controlled herself. Our focus had

to be on Daddy. Potentially, huge changes were about to come. If the neurology team decided

Daddy qualified for a shunt to deal with his hydrocephalus, it would bring about many more

questions, possible problems, and unlikely—but potential—miracles could occur.

Chapter Sixteen

FACEBOOK: August 2017

Here's how BINGO goes in a memory-care facility:
While the 'caller' is from an automated game, that doesn't mean things go smoothly.
Caller: B 12
Sylvia: B 12. No!
Bill: B-what?
Mary: 12 N
Caregiver: B 12
Caller: N 24
Sylvia: B 12 No!
Karen: She is so awful!
Bob: What?
Caller: N 24
Sylvia: No!
Michelle: [trying and failing to show Mom how fun Bingo can be] Wait. That was B 12,
     right?
Caller: G 17
Sylvia: No!
Caregiver #1: Michelle, what are you doing?
Michelle: I have no idea!
Caller: O 36
Sylvia: B 12
Bob: Ah, B 12
Mary: BINGO
Londa: No, Mary. You don't have Bingo yet.
Caller: B 45
Bill: B what?
Caller: B 45
Sylvia: B 12 No!
Trent: What are we doing?
Michelle: Bingo!
Londa: [laughing] No, Michelle.
Michelle: [ever competitive—even in memory care] Damn it!
Caregiver #2: [recapping because of Michelle and Sylvia] It's B 12, N 24, O 36
Sylvia: B 12. NO!
Caller: I 20
Sylvia: I 12. No!
Bob: Bingo!
Michelle: Damn it, Bob!

Not only did the neurology team nix the idea of a shunt, they dropped a bomb on us—Daddy had been misdiagnosed.

In an age of too many surgeons ready to whip out a knife without exploring all possibilities, some of Daddy's more classic symptoms of frontotemporal dementia (FTD) were missed. It explained his behavioral changes, the trouble he had verbalizing, and the compulsivity we had been seeing.

In a follow-up appointment at the VA, Dr. Camp reiterated the neurology team's dismissal of the normal pressure hydrocephalus diagnosis.

Michelle had agonized over the fact that Daddy had never gotten the shunt to relieve pressure on his brain after the fall. Again and again, for a year and a half, she had repeatedly questioned if we shouldn't have looked into getting the procedure done.

I always opposed it because it involved a spinal tap, during which he needed to be awake, and there was simply no way Marc Powe, as he was today, could stay still. He would rip out IVs, sutures, pull off monitors, and flip out if restrained. For me, the bad far outweighed the potential good.

But for Michelle, obsessed with the idea that he had gone untreated, not trying the procedure had bordered neglect.

Hearing that we might have put our father through an unnecessary trauma due to being erroneously diagnosed was frustrating, but liberating.

The fact that the VA and its neurology team diagnosed Daddy's FTD is a blessing. Truly, a blessing. Daddy has been diagnosed with hydrocephalus, possible Parkinson's disease, possible Agent Orange, possible strokes, and along with the correct diagnosis of FTD, he's taken thirteen blows to the head since January 2016.

"This is a good thing," I assured Michelle.

"I know. No, it is. I know. Now I can stop worrying about it." But her ace in the hole, her final hope for bringing Daddy back, was gone, and she questioned what else could have caused the FTD. Family history? Radiation from Russia? Possible exposure in Africa or the Middle East? Parkinson's?

We pondered everything— genetics, environmental factors, alcohol, and stress.

We've learned FTD is much less common than other forms of dementia, and therefore, very hard to diagnose. While people diagnosed with Alzheimer's appear to be drifting, uncertain where they are, where they are going, and/or losing concept of time, people with FTD (in the early stages) do not exhibit the same symptoms or tells and continue everyday chores, seemingly moving with purpose and intent. Thus, many misdiagnoses. Friends and family members might comment on some changes, but because a person with FTD remains fairly high functioning early on, like us, many put it off to distraction and normal "senior moments."

But there are signs.

A person with behavioral variant FTD might exhibit socially inappropriate behavior. How often did Daddy rudely interrupt conversations or blurt some odd comment out? *"It's not about me but the sixty-eight thousand soldiers who never made it home!"* We saw other indicators, such as hoarding, obsession with time, emails, "saving the world," but we didn't understand what we were looking at.

The following week, Michelle reported on her meeting with the doctor. "Dr. Camp was impressed by Daddy's intellect, even now, as characterized by Daddy's record of successful escapes from the various locked memory units. But he also kneeled in front of her a couple of times, and neither one of us knew what he wanted until he took off the nametag—mine—he was wearing and showed it to her, and she realized that he wanted to read hers, which he did. It's just amazing that a man with the amount of brain damage he has still has that kind of neurocognition."

The next day, Daddy won Bingo.

The day after that, I came into the memory care to find Daddy standing in his underwear.

The man. The myth. The memory-care legend.

On the surface, there is no hope. Not only does Mom have a disease, which will ultimately kill her, but it will also try to steal every bit of her away from us before it is done. Daddy isn't as lucky with simply having water on the brain. But deep down, we already knew that, right?

We saw it with the extreme political contributions, the belief he was talking to people at the White House, and his growing obsession with the Vietnam War. He had been forgetting words long before that. We knew. We just didn't *want* to know.

It was time to take stock of what we had going for us.

We'd never had to take the car keys away from our father. It had been escalating, but Daddy's fall had taken that hard responsibility out of our hands.

We had never had to commit either parent. Because of Daddy's condition, the hospital had only been willing to release Daddy to a memory-care facility, and then Mom had decided she wanted to be with Daddy on her own.

For me, personally, I've been mad at my dad for some time. He dumped the Power of Attorney deal in my lap with zero instruction—no details, no knowledge of who the lawyer was, or how to move on the house, car, or finances.

Financial statements were more confusing than they needed to be, but he'd made sure his long-term care with New York Life had stayed intact.

Without New York Life, I honestly don't know where we would be right now. It is the one thing he really did right, and we are so grateful. As I have said so many times, no one plans on falling and hitting their head any more than they plan on having dementia.

Mostly, however, I've been angry about the alcohol abuse. I deem it the one great flaw in his character, and it bothers me greatly as I'm his number one fan and always have been. So, how could he let me down so badly on this one? *Oh, yeah. Dementia.*

Dementia is a beast. Beyond the memory loss, the anger, the fear, and the anxiety, dementia also leads to compulsivity. New research has specifically identified frontotemporal dementia (FTD) with such behaviors,[3] and I have to wonder if that includes alcohol.

While more studies reveal heavier consumption of alcohol and its link to dementia,[4] it turns out there are also studies supporting the theory that a person who suffers from dementia might also be inclined to drink more because of the symptomology (the compulsive behaviors) of onset dementia.

In studies conducted in the United States and throughout the United Kingdom, including the National Institute of Health, FTD is thought to inhibit a person from knowing when to stop eating, drinking alcohol, or smoking.

It is no longer a question of whether Daddy's drinking brought on the dementia or the dementia brought about the heavy alcohol use. While Michelle finds comfort in knowing the promised procedure to reduce pressure from his brain wouldn't have made a difference, as his was never a hydrocephalus issue but FTD, I just get to let go.

Daddy fought many wars. He fought for world peace, for those in Third World nations who deserved better, for civil rights, for soldiers' rights, but he's never had a fair chance with FTD.

---

[3] http://www.medscape.com/viewarticle/724017
[4] https://www.healthafter50.com/memory/article/the-alarming-link-between-alcohol-and-dementia

We know in the latter stages of FTD, which is where he appears to be now, more of the brain becomes damaged. No longer isolated to the frontal portion, his diagnosis and symptoms begin sharing similarities to Mom's Alzheimer's. It's textbook behaviors. "The person may become less interested in people and things and have limited communication. They may become restless or agitated, or behave aggressively. At this late stage, they may no longer recognise friends and family, and are likely to need full-time care to meet their needs."[5]

As his FTD progresses, the symptoms are more noticeable in motor disorders. His balance and coordination are affected, as are his movements—both slow and shuffling.

Sadly, I know that in the more progressed stages, swallowing is going to become an issue.

So, here we are. Daddy has dementia. Nothing else. Mom has Alzheimer's. What are the odds both parents would, simultaneously, go down so fast but with two vastly different types of mental deterioration?

Michelle and I are genuinely grateful for the way it all happened. We got Mom and Daddy near us when we did. Uncle Stephen and Aunt Diana were able to swoop in right when I was spiraling. Michelle unearthed so many important documents for us to gain legal standing and protect our parents and their finances. Michelle was able to move in to our parents' home to protect it (and Colby). We found our parents a new home—Isle of Watercrest—with the most loving, professional, and caring staff. They are all gifts.

As the cover of this book suggests, reading about dementia and/or Alzheimer's and taking personal responsibility for your life is recommended for anyone who plans on growing old. It is a reality we all face. And in facing our particular reality, I was forced to do more soul searching about my parents. I may not understand why they did some of the things they did but what I do

---

[5]
https://www.alzheimers.org.uk/download/downloads/id/1758/factsheet_what_is_frontotemporal_dementia.pdf

know is deeply gratifying. They were progressive. They were thoughtful. They were ambassadors of tolerance and acceptance, champions of social justice, and the truest humanitarians you could ever be so fortunate to meet. They are wonderfully imperfect.

Having their legal, medical and financial issues *dumped* on us, I now see, was a gift.

I guess the only real problem I face now is…how to end this story.

As a professional writer, I have a reputation for several things. I'm funny. Okay, I know I'm not supposed to confess such things, but honestly, I crack myself up. I am also professional and, when doing a piece on another person, business, or organization, will read my notes back to them to make sure they are happy with the content. I want to be both factual and empathetic. I'm also a prolific writer.

Usually.

But with this, I have been anything but. I have fought to find the funny, and I have grieved. I have paced. I have worried. I have found study after study that, while clarifying what we saw in our parents was all part of the diagnosis, spell doom for their future.

I also write fiction and rely heavily on happy or, at the very least, satisfying finales. *How the hell am I supposed to write a happy ending to this?*

As if on cue, two great things happened.

As a writer and as a way to counter my own sadness regarding all of this, I had entered a TV pilot concept based on my father's life in an international screenwriting contest. **Spy Lies** won. I had great fun working with a producer, finely tuning the concept, and had just sent it back in when Amanda from Isle at Watercrest sent me an email. The Alzheimer's Association nearest us was looking for families to participate in the upcoming Walk to End Alzheimer's. She nominated the Powe family and urged me to call Ashley Powell in the Fort Worth office.

After several wonderful meetings with Ashley, Drew Weesner, and Liz Miller, the Powes were asked to be honorary co-chairs of the walk. They wanted us to find a family picture and share a brief bio with those who would walk to end this horrible disease.

What an honor. What an *incredible* honor.

It's a fight I know my dad would pick up in a heartbeat, Mom by his side, to do battle against.

When I told Patrick, executive director at Isle, that we were going to be the honorary chairs for the Alzheimer's Association and he playfully bowed down to me, and it struck a chord.

What if **Spy Lies** actually got picked up and became a TV show? *How flipping cool would that be?* And yet, I was, and still am, beyond humbled that my parents will be honorary chairs at the 2017 Alzheimer's Associations Walk to End Alzheimer's.

Yeah. This one matters. This really, *really* matters.

One in three seniors dies from Alzheimer's or another form of dementia. Every sixty-six seconds someone in the U.S. develops the disease, and there is no cure. Since the year 2000, deaths from heart disease have decreased by 14 percent, yet death from Alzheimer's has increased by 89 percent, but no one talks about it until it's too late!

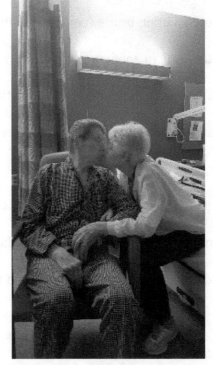

And so, I found my finale. I want this to end in a satisfying manner.

Part II of this book is a compilation of checklists we developed the hard way. I would like to think Colonel Marc Powe, a meticulous taskmaster and champion list maker, would approve. He was all about making life easier for the next guy. We hope, by sharing our mistakes and screw-ups and experiences, that will be the case for you and yours.

For the story of Marc and Karen Powe, it is not over. Not by a long shot. As we prepare to Walk to End Alzheimer's (and FTD), we created a new team page on the www.alz.org site—Our Parents Rock.

http://act.alz.org/site/TR/Walk2017/TXNorthCentralTexas?team_id=418729&pg=team&fr_id=10139

We hope you will visit and we are always taking donations.

Update: Just one week before the Walk to End Alzheimer's, my family and I had traveled some 110 miles to visit our sister-in-law for a birthday celebration. We literally pulled into the driveway when my cell phone rang. Mom had fallen, fractured her skull, broke a rib, and endured a brain bruise (complete with black eye). Michelle was unaware of this as she was in another E/R in another city with kidney stones. I would never make it back before the ambulance took her away. Remarkably, when Michelle learned what was going on (through my aggressive texting – before I knew she was also in an E/R), she checked herself out of the hospital and met Mom at a different hospital before I got there. Mom would not be able to attend the walk, nor would Michelle. It was a very unfair turn of events that have become a way of life with us. While Mom has no memory of anything, Michelle has contented herself to hearing stories of how my children pushed their papa around on the day of the walk. This really is *#LifewithDementia*.

*Please read the Postscript about our Walk to End Alzheimer's and meet some of the extraordinary women who got Daddy up on the stage!

Operation Let's End Alzheimer's!

(We're all whirling!)

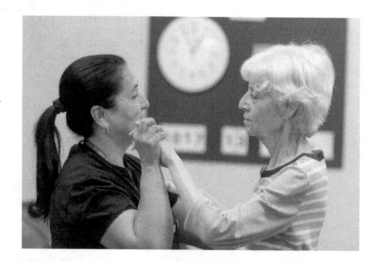

Maria L and Yaya make the best dancing partners for Mom and Daddy … If anyone could ever end Alzheimer's, it would be amazing caregivers like these women!

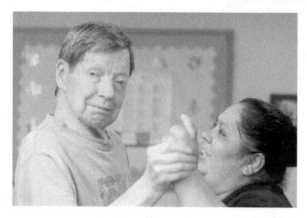

More FACEBOOK for fun:

November 2016

While shopping, Mom had three doors to consider: Men, Women, and Do Not Enter.

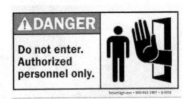

Which one do you think she picked?

November 2016

Chinese Spy?

The Setup: While cleaning out Daddy's garage, we began pulling out all his books. There were boxes and boxes of books (and we were JUST talking about Daddy's military books).
While doing so, a man pulled up and asked if we were having a garage sale.
"No! But you're welcome to any books that you'd like," we told him. We chatted, found out that he came here from China, and was trying to absorb American culture.
The Uh-Oh Moment: There is that moment when you hear, "Oooh, U.S. military strategies!" and you have to pretend you suddenly need those documents for *uh, er, um...something I forgot!*

February 2017

I Had a Dream:
I had this dream that my sister, Michelle Powe, decided to take my father and mother to Starbucks (our father LOVES coffee) AND bring their 100-lbs. dog along.
While putting Mom back in car, Daddy (who has significant brain damage) gets in the driver's seat and is READY TO GO! Mom is confused, dog is barking impatiently and Marc Powe wants the keys to crank that baby up.
hahaha... not a dream.
#glad_it_wasnt_me and #beenthere_donethat and hahahaha ... Michelle!!! Not even I would have taken the dog!!

February 2017

Post: Prison Break!

> Don't know if you all heard about the prisoner escape…it happened in Mansfield. He broke the door, decoded it or something, broke out, and an all-out search was made for him. Thank goodness, he was found lurking in the back seat of a car in the parking lot of the facility so maybe that's why it didn't make the news about MY DAD finding his way out of the memory-care center!
> YEAH, BABY!! It's hard to keep a good man down. Go, Daddy!!

February 2017

Post: Stop Thief! I mean, Daddy!

> That moment when your mom is calling another man a thief and you're looking at a watch on your father's wrist that doesn't belong to him.
> Oh, there's a thief, all right…

June 2017

> Right when you've decided that your father really can't understand what is going on around him, you look over and realize that he's reading a book— in French.

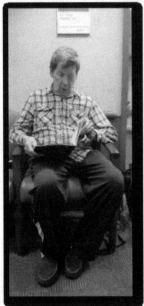

Oh, he knows. He knows…

December 2016

Post: Santa

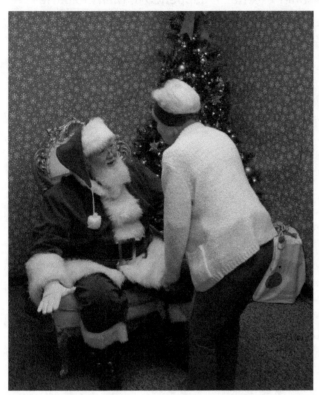

I wasn't sure about Mom meeting Santa. It could have gone one of two ways…and she was a bit overwhelmed and hung back. When we lured her forward Santa understood instantly…
He said, "I remember you when you were a little girl," and Mom lit up.
"Santa!"
THAT was my Christmas present! She didn't want to leave him.
To Judge Fite Century 21 and the BEST real estate agent EVER—Sarah Ervin Padgett—thank you for transporting us back in time to a happy place with a light heart, big dreams, and hope. I know it was "just" your office but for us—for me—it was the closest to the North Pole as I've ever been and my heart will never be the same. Other businesses might say, "Merry Christmas," but you made it happen. xxoo

April 2017

Post: Elvis Lives

We are standing in the memory-care facility when a woman rolls up to Robb Allred on her wheelchair and tells him he's "tall like Elvis Presley."
He joked "but not as good looking."
Oh, she wasn't having that and commented on his "red" beard.
(note: Extreme twitching by Robb) He later regretted truly that when she complimented him he didn't do a lip curl to say, "Thank ya, thank ya vury much." Robb said "Dang it. I want a do-over."
Robb—it's a memory-care center. We can go back in 20 minutes and play that whole scene over again and no one else will remember!

April 2017

Post: Shirt Off My Back!

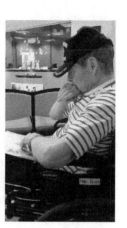

Took my parents to the doctor today. It went like this:
Mom was in a loop.
Mom: Who's glasses are these?
Alex: Those are yours.
Mom: They're mine?
...
Mom: Who's glasses are these?
Alex: Those are yours.
Mom: They're mine?
...again and again but I didn't mind because I really needed Mom to NOT notice that Daddy was wearing her shirt.
We were almost done when...her eyes kind of squinted.
Mom: Is that my shirt?!?!
Alex: Wha?? Noooooooooo! Oh, don't be absurd! Daddy could never wear one of your shirts! (Yeah. That's your favorite shirt, Mom and might I say...he's wearing it well).
Uncertain, she went along with it...in the car:
Mom: Who's glasses are these?
Daddy: Ohh. [and he reached over and put them on!]

May 2017

POST: Mean Girl Table

Ever been in on a gossip session at a memory-care facility? It goes like this:
Resident 1: I don't like that person. I don't even know if it's a man or a woman.
Resident 2: I don't know either.
Alex (laughing): Holy cow, you two! She's a woman!
Resident 1 (looking snottily at Alex [trying to decide if *she's* a man or woman]): Well. Then. It should try to look like one.
Resident 2: Are you sure it's a woman?
Alex: Wow. This is a tough crowd. Why don't you like her?
Resident 1: She hops.
Resident 2: And she steals food. All the time she steals food.
Alex: Well, she needs the extra calories for all that hopping.
Resident 1: Well, *it* should stop hopping.
#LifeInMemoryCare and #Alexisawoman—fyi

April 2017

Post: Window Protocol

> New policy at the memory-care facility. All windows must be locked at all times and…if opened, can only be opened about 4 inches.
> I say, "Uh. Please tell me this doesn't have anything to do with my father." But I knew better. Oh, I knew better. "So, what's Jason Bourne up to now?" I ask.
> Understanding that his own bedroom window had been locked up tight, Agent Bourne, aka—my father—gathered up a pair of shoes, broke into another resident's room, opened her window and threw his shoes out the window.
> Then, skulking backward, he hid behind the door when a caregiver came in.
> He was busted by the room's resident who watched the entire exchange.
> I asked, "What? Why do you think he did that?"
> Caregiver: He wanted shoes for when he breaks out again.

April 2017

POST: Operation Move Patio Furniture

> I went to the memory-care facility to find much of the staff standing at the big window by the dining room, smiling. We looked out.
> There he was. My dad. Moving at the warp speed of a drowsy turtle, lifting up heavy patio furniture, and rearranging all the chairs and tables. [Shuffle, shuffle, move, move]
> I had to ask. "You don't mind him moving all that around?"
> They said, "What's the point? You can't stop him."
> Indeed.

May 2017

POST: They'll Let Anyone In

> Michelle Powe (sister) gets a call at 11:45 pm from memory-care facility who can't calm Mom down. She is almost hysterical, telling Michelle that she and our dad have been taken hostage. Mom doesn't know what "the people" have done with her husband, and Michelle MUST jump in her car and drive to save them!
> After a few more minutes…
> Michelle (flustered/exhausted): Well. Where is Daddy now?
> Mom: Oh, he's right here with me [she forgot about the hostage thing]
> We tag-team and I go to see her the next day. I am prepared for hostage talk and have it all planned out…but she reversed it on me.

She is stunned to see me as they are not letting people IN.
Mom: How did you get in here?
Alex: Well, I...(I pause. This could be a trap. But how?) I...walked in?
She looks around, sneaky-like. Mom: You're lucky. They don't let people in here.
Alex: Who?
Mom: I don't know. Undesirable people, I guess.
Alex: Oh. well. I guess we know they like us then, huh?
[pause]
Mom: How did you get in?
Heyyyy, wait a minute. What's she saying there?

May 2017

POST: Night Shift

Hey, EVERYONE...my dad got a job. Yep. Yep. It's true. Turns out that memory-care facilities have to a quarterly fire drills. You know, make sure everyone exits properly, protocol is in place. And...as the manager explained to me..." Thanks to your father, we don't just do quarterly fire drills, we do monthly!"
And the nurse says, "Sometimes more!"
Isn't that great?? The old man found himself a purpose after all.
You're welcome, everyone...you're welcome.

October 2017

POST: What's Clothes, Anyway?

My dad gives new meaning to the saying, "Keep your pants on!"

September 2017

POST: Where's the Colonel?

At what point do we all get tired of asking this question??? Where isn't he? He's the man, the myth, the memory care legend!

May 2017

POST: Are you my mother?

> Well...I just got a text message from the event coordinator at the memory-care facility and...my dad just proposed to her.
> Two huge problems:
> 1. When my mom finds out about this ... oh, baby!
> 2. I ain't callin' her mom!

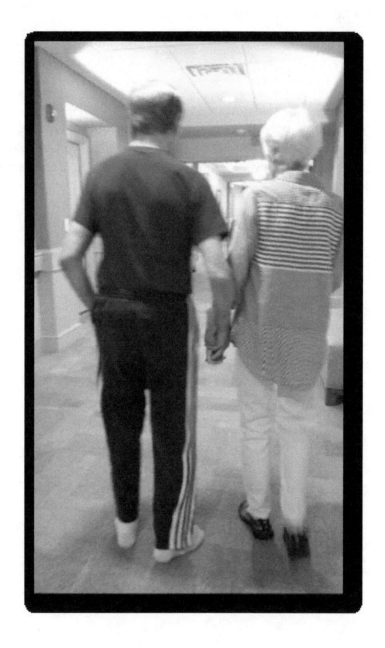

Mom and Daddy Making the Rounds

June 2017

You've heard of using a file to break out of jail...yeah. Last night our dad was extremely "active." There was a fight, threat of police and Michelle Powe ran up there...
her early Father's present to her dad?
Yeah. She gave him a file.
Okay, an emery board but it's still a file.
Nice work, Michelle.
Go for it, Daddy. FILE AWAY at that door!
Happy Father's Day.

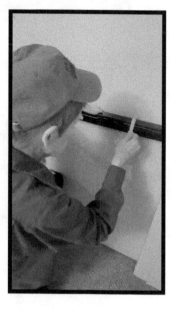

June 2017

...that moment when you are in Half Price Books and your mother—very confused and frail—blurts out that she is homeless and everyone looks at you like you're stealing from this tiny, sweet person.

November 2016

Got to take Mom to vote! Having a voice is so important!

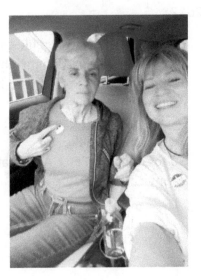

June 2017

POST: Lock-Down

> ...and the caregivers say, "There is no way he could get into any of the rooms because the doors are locked," yet our father is nowhere to be found in the memory care, and so there is a door-to-door search for the man who was trained in covert operations...and he is eventually found in a room that was LOCKED and other caregivers say, "Oh, yes, 'I've seen him pick the locks.'"...and he was then found uncoiling a wire hanger...because he's got allllllllllll night to figure this out!

July 2017

POST: Mom's Favorite Shirt #LifewithDementia

> Michelle took my mom out for lunch and to get her nails done...when they got back, they found my dad trying on all my mom's T-shirts.
> Err...what'cha doin' there, Daddy?
> (Please don't let it be the red and white striped shirt...please don't let it be the red and white striped shirt...please don't let it be the red and white striped shirt...)
> Man...we gotta get Daddy a striped shirt and fast!

August, 2017

POST: The Peach and the Donut

Part I: Just Peachy—How Alzheimer's Steals Appetite but It Didn't Count on a Burger Tree

It's vital that Mom eats so I promised good times and lunch. She was pretty confused today so medicine was imperative, making food imperative.

She wanted a burger.

Excellent.

But as soon as she got it, she refused to eat.

I begged and pleaded but to no avail.

Frustrated with me, she waved a hand out the window. "I would rather eat that tree."

"That tree? Well, that tree looks delicious!"

She looked at me.

"Or what about that tree? Or that one? Yummy!" She kind of laughed, so…"Oooh, look at that delicious one!" and when we turned into a neighborhood, I threw the car into park, jumped out, snapped a twig off the tree, and handed it to Mom. "Look at this morsel."

She laughed.

As I continued to point out all the delicious trees I would totally eat…I saw it. A peach tree! Someone had a peach tree in their front yard. Peach theft!! I grabbed one and ran back, presenting—no, daring her to eat it.

She said, "Well, that doesn't look very appealing."

Look. Lady. It's 102 degrees outside. Work with me. I snagged her burger and ran off to another tree, ripped off some leaves, wrapped them around the burger as I ran back and handed it to her…

Did she believe? Did she buy it? Did she believe I stumbled upon a burger tree? Would she be convinced?

She said, "If I eat this, will you please stop?"

(But I can't! I just can't!)

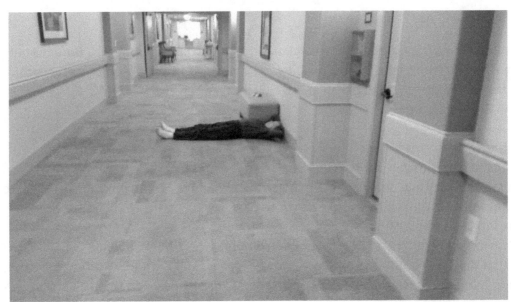

Part II: Just Peachy—How Dementia Can Give Too BIG of an Appetite and Really Bring a Fella Down

When we got back to the memory-care facility, we found him…laid out.

Earlier I brought (the best!) donuts from DONUT TIME in Waxahachie and handed them out to everyone.

Tall Bill (not to be confused with Older Bill), Sylvia, Dot, Bob, and others happily picked out a fave donut.

Because Trent, a known thief and donut hoarder was asleep, Daddy (a known thief and donut hoarder) went to town on the rest of the box…then he went down.

Full belly…now he's jelly.

October 8, 2017
POST: Walk to End Alzheimer's Reality Check

Funny line of the day? A man bopped over to Kyle and asked, "What country are we in?"

Kyle: The United States?
Man: Okay, good

And away he went … *You, sir, are in the right place!* I guess if you have dementia/Alzheimer's today would have seemed like a crazy day.

To clarify the sea of flowers: Orange means you are a caregiver; purple means you lost a loved one to Alzheimer's; yellow means you have a loved one with the disease and blue means you are diagnosed with it.

August 2017

POST: Operation Write

> Mom said she "can't do anything anymore..." so I suggested we write some letters to some friends. She couldn't write letters so...okay...let's do the envelopes, and I'll write the letter
> She agreed.
> She couldn't understand how to properly fill out an envelope and the struggle was mighty but today...my mom was mightier and she conquered it!!!

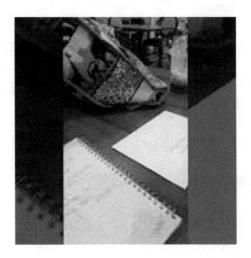

Mom writing vs. Alzheimer's

August 2017

"It is Day 210 of my incarceration and my captors appear impervious to my attempts to distract and evade. I have pulled fire alarms, moved furniture, broken out windows, locked doors, and escaped through others only to be foiled at each turn. I have stolen personal property, written cryptic notes, and flooded the shower. Now it is time to take it up a notch..."

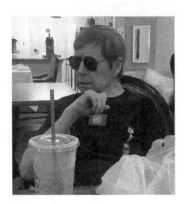

Once a super spy .... Always a super spy

August 2017

POST: To the Bank We Go!

Took parents to the bank for an outing.

Mom has a recurring fear of having no money so I pre-arranged for the bank tellers to tell her that they were watching her money. We cashed a check and the teller handed a $10 bill to Mom. This adventure took over three hours, required two apple pies, two small cokes, and the repeated phrase of, "I promise, Mom, you have money in the bank," no less than 37 times.

As our adventure drew to an end, I promised Mom that "I've got you. Don't worry. You have money in your bank account," and she said, "Well, what does that have to do with anything we've been talking about?"

Well, it ... uh ... [she's forgotten! abort! abort!] Alex: Nothing. I was just kind of, ya know, babbling. How's that apple pie?

Mom: What apple pie?

Alex: That...what the heck? Where is it? [sees Daddy eating BOTH apple pies at exact time]

Mom: Well, at some point, we need to talk about finances. I am very worried about money.

Alex: DADDY!!

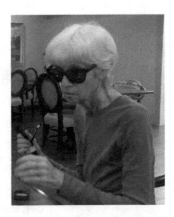

Mom doesn't know she's not a super spy ... or maybe it is we who don't know. Wasn't it Mom who got some classified pictures?

Who are you, Karen Powe? Who are you?

August 2017

POST: Another Break-in or Break-Out?

Is this random? Is this Marc?

We get to the table in the dining hall and its full on. Trent is fighting with one of the caregivers about his food, Ms. Mary wants her food now, Mom has mistaken her napkin for her hamburger and is attempting to eat it, Joan, pants less, is crying at the threshold of the dining area, and one of the new gentlemen (don't know his name yet) has a few choice words about his food. Someone has put Lil' Rascals on in the activity room and it's too loud. Ms. Sylvia is yelling back at the noisy sounding children in the next room. "No!" and "No, you will not." "No! You will not!" It is complete pandemonium and...and...

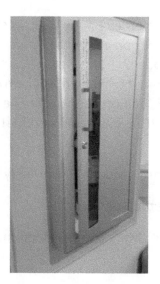

You know that one kid who is ALWAYS the problem and yet, amidst the chaos ... look at him eating so quietly and happily. Really, Marc? Who ... oh, but who is the one who jimmied open the lock to the fire extinguisher before I came around the corner to catch him???

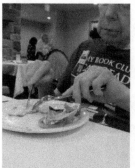

HMMMM, DADDY? Hmmm??
  And what do you do with a plastic blue cup when you come across one? Why ... you crush it, slide it up and down in the door jam in hopes of popping open the door when no one is looking.

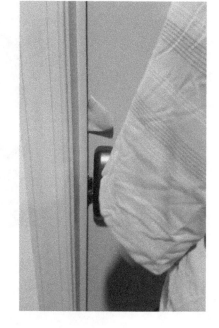

Unfortunately for you, Colonel, sir, you taught your daughters
a little too well ...

Step away from the cup, sir. Step away from the cup.

September 2017:

Yesterday Daddy took his clothes off (in the patio area) and hung his shirt on a tree and his pants on a branch.
Today?
Round two...he tried the trees and bein' free in the breeze again but...alas...the caregivers put his belt on backward so he couldn't get his pants off.
CURSE YOU, CAREGIVERS!! Foiled again!

This is Mom's Shirt, Daddy!!

September 2017:

Got Mom a new striped shirt:

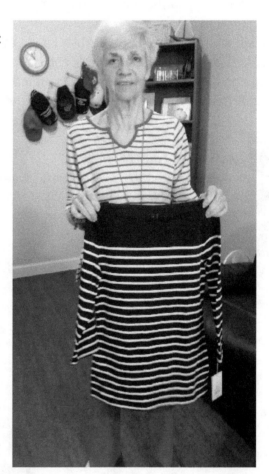

PART II

Operation Checklists

One day, Michelle, Mom, and I were standing in the kitchen of the memory-care facility when one of the residents known for such activities began dropping his pants and exposing himself.

Mom rolled her eyes and said to Michelle, "Watch out. I've seen this before."

Chapter Seventeen

FACEBOOK: *April 2017*

> *I was working out at the gym this morning when a message came in from the memory care that there had been another escape attempt, and I suddenly realized…this is why I work out! One day, I, too, will torture my own children and they will get random calls and texts. "She's escaped again!" and "She's bustin' out windows again!"*
> *Look alive, my sweet children. I have a plan now and your future has never looked so busy!*
> *#OperationPaybacks*

Prior to the publication of this book, I asked several members of my Silver Sneakers class to read and comment on its content. Collectively, they are an amazing group of highly social, active, savvy seniors who have already or are in the process of creating their own Power of Attorney and Executor of Will appointees, including medical, financial, and funeral arrangements. Yet all were surprised by much information is provided in this chapter. What you eat, how you live, if you exercise, even how you laugh, has a direct impact on your health as you age. The correlation between these things and increased risks of dementia deserve serious consideration.

It would be absurd—even negligent—to state by simply changing your lifestyle habits you will be free of Alzheimer's and dementia risks. However, by taking a more proactive approach to your own life you can ensure greater odds in your favor; you will become healthier and, hopefully, more independent. Positive lifestyle changes can increase mood, production, allow for better sleep, and greater peace of mind. What research shows us is that these positive attributes do help guard against or decrease chances of the disease, and by not taking a more proactive stance in your own future, you are accepting your current situation and/or your own fears.

The following are some small but important changes you can make in your own life.

Where Are You Right Now?

A surprising study by Bank of America Merrill Lynch (2017) revealed that workers aged 21 to 34 are the most likely to contribute salary to a 401(k) plan, followed by workers aged 35 to 49. The group least likely to contribute are those who are the closest in age to retirement. Workers aged 50 to 68 contribute the least.

According to the Economic Policy Institute, nearly half of those in the 50 to 68 population do not have a retirement nest egg. In fact, most are actually in debt. More worrisome, a significant number of those soon-to-be retirees believe that social security will provide enough income for them to "get by."[6] In actuality, social security, on average, pays approximately $1,360 per month, or $16,320 annually.

Did you know that it costs the average healthy 65-year-old couple $400,000 (or more) in medical costs, *not* including long-term care? And while you may not yet be ready for long-term care, it will be the single most important gift you give your family and yourself. No one ever plans on having dementia, being inflicted with cancer, or face-planting on his kitchen floor.

The good news is, with 401(k)s and generous annual contribution limits, it is never too late. According to financial experts, workers in their fifties and early sixties can plump up their own 401(k) and retirement fund for the future.

Learning to curb needless spending is imperative.

Another study shows that millennials are the most in debt and most stressed working group. While they may be savvy about insurance and 401(k) plans, they make more impulsive buys than any other group—and they are paying for it. According to both *Money* and *Business Insider* magazines, the top ten I-Want-It-Now purchases lean toward craft brews, tattoos and piercings,

---

[6] https://www.fool.com/careers/2017/08/06/study-millennials-are-poor-and-work-obsessed.aspx

charity donations at the cash register, energy drinks and/or expensive coffeehouse drinks, leisurewear, same-day delivery, exotic pets (and their needs), and gas station food, in addition to fast food and great—yet expensive—data plans for their phones.

As you plan for your future, take time to talk to your children and grandchildren about their own lifestyle and spending habits. By getting your own affairs in order and speaking to family about it, you are also educating your loved ones about their own future.

In her lifetime, the average woman spends a stunning amount of money on things that have no value for her future and welfare. Money spent on makeup, clothes, hair, and cosmetic surgery are hard to total up knowing this is money forever lost and will never help the greatest moments of financial need.

Average annual costs:

❖ Makeup = $15,000.00
❖ Clothes = $3,000.00
❖ Hair stylist = $1,400.00
❖ Hair products = $600.00
❖ Manicurist = $1,300.00

In 2014, the cosmetic surgery was a $13.6 billion-dollar industry in just one year with most sales generated from breast enhancements, facial reconstruction, and weight management procedures. According to a CBS report, the average monthly cost for a faithful Dunkin' Donuts, Starbucks, or Caribou Coffee customer is $65, and $780 annually. That's good money gone that is never coming back.

There is no magical advice to be offered here beyond…don't do that.

The point is highlighting expenses we think so little of and/or we justify. We are all guilty of making frivolous purchases, but we can no longer afford (quite literally) to ignore one glaring reality—if that money had been saved rather than spent, how much more financially secure would you be now?

Ah, but it's too late, right? No sense crying over spilled mocha lattes.

Not quite.

There are things that can be done right now to help you and your loved ones later on when critically important financial, legal, medical, and emotional decisions need to be made.

- *How are you living fiscally?*
- *How are you living physically?*
- *How are you living nutritionally?*
- *How are you living emotionally?*

How Are You Living Fiscally?

Define what financial independence/success means to you. This is a strategy that financial advisors always use to get clients thinking about their own future. More specifically, how to get their clients to take action for their own future. Most people are afraid to make the changes needed to ensure greater financial stability and so…they simply don't make the change. Perhaps you already have independence.

You are ready to implement a plan. Otherwise, you need to know both current and future costs for independent living. This means gathering information.

- ❖ Assisted and/or memory-care living
- ❖ Current medication costs
- ❖ Current bills, including home mortgage or rental, utilities, credit card, auto, auto insurance, medical insurance, credit cards, and any other outstanding debt to creditors, banks, institutions, education and/ family and friends
- ❖ Possess a realistic picture of your finances
  - ➢ Know your own bank statements
  - ➢ Understand any 401(k)s, IRAs, CDs, stocks, bonds, and any other investments you or your family may have
  - ➢ Understand what you owe on your mortgage or how your rent might be affected in the future if you were sick or incapacitated. How will this affect others?

How Are You Living Physically?

While there are no guarantees to hold off Alzheimer's or other forms of dementia any more than there are any guarantees for a long, healthy life, regular exercise can improve your chances. In fact, regular exercise is the most reliable, cost-effective, long-term solution for better health. Active lifestyles can lower risk of heart disease, stroke, type-2 diabetes, some cancers, depression, and dementia. But there is growing evidence exercise can reduce the risk of mental illness and allow seniors to potentially remain independent much longer in life.

Researchers from the Annals of Internal Medicine found that people who were physically fit in their forties and fifties were almost 40 percent less likely to develop Alzheimer's/dementia by their mid-sixties compared to those who did not exercise. And into those later years, another study found that regular exercise helped to reduce risk of dementia-related deaths.

So, how active are you? What can you do?

Exercises for seniors:

> **Endurance**: Walking, jogging (though this higher-impact activity can cause joint/back issues), dancing, or swimming. A minimum of 150 minute of exercise per week is recommended, however, go slowly. If you are not active, begin with a low- to no-impact activity, such as swimming, for approximately 10 minutes and slowly build.

> **Strength training**: Perhaps the most feared, yet important, kind of training is strength (weight) training. It is recommended weight workouts, which include machines, free weights, and resistance bands, take place two or three times a week. You should work your shoulders, arms, chest, back, hips, and legs. Begin with light weights and gradually grow as your muscles do. It is highly recommended to meet with a personal trainer to

begin a safe routine. Proper form and posture are extremely important to minimize risk of injury. The benefits of weight training for seniors is tremendous!

Do not start any activity without consent from your primary physician. Do find a personal trainer who has experience working with seniors. Healthways and Tivity Health are two training programs that train instructors specializing in working with the older population.

Balance: Balance is the key to everything in your day-to-day living, and how you function safely and efficiently. There are many reasons for poor balance, from inner ear disturbances, poor nutrition, allergies, and sleep deprivation to neurological and/or developmental conditions or previous injuries. An imbalance can greatly affect how you walk, step, lift, even sit. Poor balance translates to alignment issues with your physical being and decreased abilities. In short, balance is everything. By working with a personal trainer or instructor, you can develop a great sense of independence and strength through better balance.

Stretch and Relaxation: Great flexibility, through stretch and relaxation movement, can provide greater range of motion and reduce risk of injury. It may also increase balance.

Again, please speak with your physician first and make your intentions what kind of exercise you hope to participate in clear then find the right class and/or instructor to work with you. Start slowly, be smart, and have fun.

As a Silver Sneakers certified instructor, I promise the social aspect of group training cannot be undervalued. I highly recommend group classes offering endurance, strength, and balance training with stretching in a forty-five-minute format that fits all fitness levels.

Today, advances in technology and a greater emphasis on cross-disciplinary research helps further our understanding of how motor skills are learned and controlled. We are learning that functional movement, motor development, and fitness are not independent of one another but all work together to make for better, healthier lives for people of all ages.

In the September 2017 World Congress on Neurology conference in Kyoto, Japan, yet another study linked the importance of being physically fit and cognitive activity as a deterrent to dementia. The study, involving 1,700 participants, shows that staying physically fit and keeping your brain fit can help stave off dementia.

How Are You Living Nutritionally?

Most of us exceed the daily recommendations for added sugars, sodium, and saturated fats, which explains why Americans are also more likely to be diagnosed with more than one chronic condition in their lifetime. Some of the most common diagnoses are arthritis, heart disease, asthma, high blood pressure, and diabetes.[7] More problematic is the fact that the United States has more overweight and obese citizens than any other country, with 70.9 percent of men and 61.9 percent of women compared to 38 percent of men and 36.9 percent of women worldwide.

As science links nutrition to Alzheimer's and other forms of dementia, it comes as no surprise to learn Alzheimer's and dementia rates are lowest in African, India, and South Asia and highest in Western Europe, the United States, and growing exponentially in Japan and China. All nations where food, food development, and preparation have changed.

Why?

Historically speaking, diets worldwide were previously based in vegetable products and natural grains and fewer animal products. But in countries where diet has changed so, too, has the human form and health. Using Japan as an example, traditional diets were rice-based with rationed meats. From 1961 to 2008, however, meat and animal fat consumption markedly increased. Documented cases of Alzheimer's disease increased as well. A similar conclusion was drawn in China.[8]

As we introduce "fake" foods into our diet, we jeopardize our own health. Perhaps some of the most dangerous foods for brain and physical health are hydrogenated foods, including

---

[7] Fox, M. United States Comes in Last Again on Health, Compared to Other Countries, Health, NBC News, November 16, 2016.

[8] Greger, M., M.D., Where Are the Lowest Rates of Alzheimer's in the World?, Nutritional Fact. www.nutritionalfacts.org. November 12, 2015.

margarine (instead of real butter), vegetable shortening, packaged snacks, and pre-packaged frozen meals, baked goods of the premade variety, ready-to-use dough, fried foods, and coffee creamers, as well as sugar substitutes and high fructose corn syrup.

When it comes to proper digestion and health in regards to food consumption, one of the most recent interruptions is the so-called "new" grain. Strictly for purposes of profit and more expedient production, techniques have been revised in grain processing. Those techniques strip the more nutritious components of the grain (bran and germ) that leads to faster spikes in blood sugars and changes the digestion process. When you read labels stating flour has been *enriched* or *bleached* you should understand the grain was nutritionally stripped then chemically re-enriched for nutritional purposes.

The old adage, "You are what you eat," has never been more true.

The human body is *not* designed to digest genetically modified, nutritionally stripped wheat. Just as it is unable to breakdown and process chemical-based drinks in a healthy way, the body is also unable to beneficially process this new wheat, and we are seeing the results.

Nutritionally speaking, just as with anyone else, the recommendations those diagnosed with Alzheimer's or dementia are simple:

- ❖ Maintain a balanced diet of vegetables, fruits, while grain (not bleached, enriched, processed, etc.), low-fat dairy products. and lean protein foods
- ❖ Limit high saturated fats and cholesterol
- ❖ Stay away from hydrogenated foods
- ❖ Limit added sugar
- ❖ Cut back on high sodium and use less salt

How Are You Living Emotionally?

Are you depressed?

Do you feel anxious?

Are you an introvert who shies away from social settings?

Do you tend to lean toward more neurotic behaviors?

The answers to these questions are important as more and more research indicates a connection between depression and neuroticism and increased risks of dementia.

First, to be clear, *neuroticism* is a life-long or long-term trait manifesting in the form of a more negative, more pessimistic outlook. People with this condition tend to show signs of depression, self-imposed worry, guilt, self-deprecation, anger, envy, and anxiety than others. Those who suffer from neurotic tendencies are more likely to be in debt, have cosmetic surgery, contemplate or attempt suicide, and be more introverted in social settings.

In what researchers are describing as "the clearest evidence to date linking depression and dementia," there is some positive news. In a study conducted by the neuropsychology department of Rush University, in Chicago, they have discovered one of the early signs or symptoms of dementia is depression. According to the Alzheimer's Association, nearly 40 percent of people with Alzheimer's disease also experience depression.

Yet another study conducted in a neuropsychology clinic through the Morris Psychological Group out of New Jersey, the damage that long-term depression does to the brain may lead to dementia.

One of the more optimistic studies at the University of Texas Medical School reveals there is hope. If people pursue medical treatment for their depression, thus helping improve memory, concentration, decision-making, and mood, it could also reduce the risk for dementia.[9]

The Weight of Stress on Your Mind

A study in Sweden specifically looked at women to measure levels of anxiety and stress. The results revealed those who scored highest on a test for neuroticism were twice as likely to develop Alzheimer's than women with lower scores. Further, the study found that extroverted women experienced less long-term stress, allowing researchers to hypothesize that those subjects had reduced risks of dementia. Theoretic conclusion? Those who are most neurotic and least social have the highest risk for Alzheimer's disease. It is not just neurotic behavior that increase the risks of Alzheimer's but also chronic stress, as it brings about a host of health issues, including negative impact on brain function.

A study on laboratory rats revealed that long-term stress causes short-term memory loss and eventual long-term memory impairment. Stress can actually age the brain, altering the grooves in the brain pattern and changing both behavior and health of the brain.[10]

The Weight on Your Heart

At the XXI World Congress of Neurology in Vienna, 2013, a team of researchers from Argentina presented findings on stress and possible triggers for the onset of Alzheimer's, specifically emotional stress brought on by trauma. Researchers found that 72 percent, that is nearly three out

---

[9] Bowers, Elizabeth S., Depression as a Risk Factor for Dementia, https://www.everydayhealth.com/news/depression-risk-factor-dementia/

[10] Johansson, L., X Gue, PR Duberstein, "Midlife Personality and Risk of Alzheimer Disease and Distress: A 38-Year Follow-Up," Neurology. October 21, 2014; 83(17); 1538-44. doi: 10.1212/WNL.0000000000000907Epub 2014 Oct 1.

of every four, of Alzheimer's patients had experienced severe emotional trauma two years prior to their diagnosis. Such traumas include:

- ❖ The death of a spouse, partner, or child
- ❖ Victim of a crime, particularly a violent crime such as assault or robbery
- ❖ Car accident
- ❖ Financial trouble, including "pension shock"
- ❖ Diagnosis of a severe illness of a family member or close loved one[11]

Whether you have been diagnosed with dementia or you're a caregiver for someone with the diagnosis, the need to care for your emotional, physical, and financial wellbeing are crucial.

Some proactive steps you can take:

- ❖ Make a change in your diet. Talk to your doctor and find an expert if you are unsure of how to make those changes or what to do.
- ❖ Ramp up your fitness goals!
- ❖ Get social. Refocus your efforts on communal and/or charitable works. Get involved with your church or local politics. Set luncheon dates with friends or, better yet, start a walking club.
- ❖ Take care of your money. Start asking more questions about your finances. Perhaps you are the person who pays all the bills in your home. It is time to share your knowledge. In doing this, you can flex your financial knowledge and memory muscles but also ensure that things can and will be taken care of if or when you are otherwise incapacitated.

There are a few things to keep in mind as you choose specialists to assist you on your way to a healthy body. A *nutritionist* typically holds an undergraduate or graduate degree in nutrition and works as a research scientist or as a health and wellness educator. Many claiming to be nutritionists have very little training, no degree, and/or are selling nutrition products rather than offering research-based, safe advice, so do the extra legwork and investigate!

---

[11] "Stress Related to Alzheimer's Clinical Onset," September 30, 2013,
http://www.medicalnewstoday.com/releases/266702.php

A *Registered Dietician Nutritionist* (RDN) is a nutritionist accredited by the Academy of Nutrition and Dietetics (formerly known as the American Dietetic Association or ADA). An RDN has complete an undergraduate program in nutrition and also a one-year clinical internship program and may only maintain registered status with continued education, certifications, and training. Verify the credentials of the RDN or nutritionist you speak with before following any plan and always share your information with your primary physician to stay safe.

The difference between personal trainers and fitness instructors varies as well. Neither one requires a college degree, which is a true failing on the part of the industry. However, very qualified trainers and instructors are out there. It's up to you to be selective.

Fitness instructors must have group certification but may also specialize in specific classes such as Silver Sneakers, Zumba, aqua, or spinning. Even if you take a specialized class, be sure the instructor possesses a group certification in addition to the single specialized class. That ensures greater knowledge about functional movement, muscle groups, and how to safely train and move.

Personal trainers, on the other hand, must go through a far more intensive program covering details on the human anatomy, principals of wellness and fitness, and kinesiology (the study of movement).

When it comes to trainers, the fitness industry has all shapes and sizes. The world of online certification expands that world exponentially and allows for those with limited education and little practical experience. Don't be afraid to ask questions! Ask to see their résumé. Make sure you find a trainer well versed in human anatomy and kinesiology, preferably a trainer with a bachelor's or master's degree in kinesiology. This is your health we're talking about, after all.

In the next chapters, you will be shown more ways to be proactive with your future, how to help family members maintain some measure of control if or when dementia enters your lives. While the disease is debilitating, we must continue to fight it in any way we can. This includes maintaining control of our personal and professional lives.

"Anything good for your heart is good for your brain."

-Laura Boxley, PhD
Assistant Professor of Clinical Psychiatry
Ohio State University, Columbus

Chapter Eighteen

Mom: I should probably go to the bank.
Alex: Okay. What do you need?
Mom: [looking incredulous] I need money.
Alex: Well, yeah. Sure. But is there something in particular you need?
Mom: Money.
Alex: Well, I've got this. [handed her a $10 that I knew she was going to immediately
*   lose and planned on stealing it back once she forgot about it]*
Mom: What's this for?
Alex: For you. You said you needed money.
Mom: I did?
Alex: Yeah. Just now. You were saying that you needed some money.
Mom: Well, I don't want to take your money. What I need to do is go to the bank.
Alex: I really feel like we've covered this...
Mom: We have?
Alex: Yeah. I'm really feeling like—
Mom: [noticing her $10 bill] What's this?
Alex: Yup. Yup. We've definitely covered this before.

As I began to get things under control (thanks in part to those I refer to as Team Powe), I met

with a field officer from Veterans Affairs in regards to additional funds my father was entitled to

help off-set additional living costs that come with memory care and his increased number of

medications. Remarkably, after more than thirty years in the military, nearly being killed

countless times, and obtaining crucial intelligence information for our nation's security, he

qualified for exactly $408.97 each month.

"I'll take it!" I said.

Shameful, I know, but that four hundred plus a month helps with bills and fighting the VA is an

exhaustive, time-consuming, infuriating exercise in futility designed purely to make a loved one

spend their life on hold, bouncing from one department to another without every really getting an

answer, all in an effort to redesign the entire U.S. government infrastructure.

It seemed much easier just saying 'yes' to what sounded more like chump change and calling it a day.

But I wasn't done yet.

I had to wait for a letter approving me as Daddy's fiduciary appointee in the mail then go to the bank and open an entirely new account in just Marc Powe and Alexandra Allred's names, titled a *Federal Fiduciary Account*, that would allow for direct deposit only.

Really? I looked at my otherwise super-sweet field officer. "Really?"

Really.

All too often the VA is contacted by an individual caregiver, or worse, a memory-care facility, to inform them the veteran is going to be displaced from his or her residence because two or more months have passed without the facility or caregiver receiving payment. The VA, however, has cut the check and sent it out to the appointed family member for proper payment. Instead, of it going where it's meant to, the family member or long-term care appointee simply pockets the money—veteran be damned.

I learned from other caregivers, administrators in assisted-living and memory-care facilities, and insurance agents these stories are not at all isolated but more commonplace that anyone wants to believe. And it is information like this that enrages and saddens me. It also makes me more understanding of financial, medical, and living institutions as we deal with seniors. Supposed loved ones and caregivers are stealing from our seniors in epic proportions.

As Power of Attorney, my agenda is simple. I try to imagine WWMD—*Operation What Would Marc Do?*

I have no idea how long my parents will live. I have no idea what medical situations or emergencies might come up. I cannot guess what costs lay ahead. So, I manage every penny I can.

The last section offered changes for the present. This section prepares you for the future, when you can no longer make important decisions for yourself. Ironically, while this is all about you, your decisions today have a huge impact on others tomorrow.

Think about it—

- ❖ *What legal plans have you made?*
  - ➢ *Do you have a living will?*
  - ➢ *Do you have a Power of Attorney?*
  - ➢ *Have you specified any donations or special instructions to your church, minister, favorite charity or organization?*
- ❖ *What's your healthcare plan?*
  - ➢ *Do you have health insurance? Long-Term Care?*
  - ➢ *Does your doctor understand your long-term medical plans?*
  - ➢ *Do family members know what medications you take or what your medical history looks like? Would they know who to call?*
- ❖ *What's your team roster look like?*
  - ➢ *Do your relatives and friends know who your Power of Attorney is?*
  - ➢ *Do your relatives and friends know who your physician is?*
  - ➢ *Are your friends and family aware of who your neighbors are and could they get in touch with them if needed?*

Do you have the answers? Most of us don't. Michelle and I certainly didn't before we began this journey. To avoid a lot of the wasted time, energy, and frustration we went through, I've provided a few helpful tips we picked up along the way that might help you find your own answers.

What Legal Plans Have You Made?

The questions are 'do you have a living will,' 'do you have a power of attorney,' and 'have you specified any donations or special instructions to your church, favorite charity, or organization?' The purpose of the will is for you to have the final say in how you want things to be taken care of and how you want any money, property, and possessions to be disbursed. But because the idea of writing out your last wishes is so uncomfortable; most people simply avoid doing so. In fact, over 60 percent of Americans do not have a will.

Have you ever wondered what happens if someone dies and they do not have a will?

If you die without a will, your estate enters into what is termed *Law of Intestacy*. This mean the state where you live (and all states have different laws) will determine who your heirs are and how your possessions and monies are distributed. The state will also choose who will act as the executor of your estate. While spouses typically stand at the top of the list, followed by children, followed by surviving parents, each case can be different. Unmarried partners, friends, and charities do not make the list at all.

Unlike wills, people tend to be more proactive about their Power of Attorney. According to the American Association of Retired Persons (AARP), over half the adults in the U.S. have a Power of Attorney named. The reason for this is not so much for concern of their estate but health care. This health-care Power of Attorney grants the POA legal authority to make those difficult decisions in the event you are otherwise incapacitated.

As you have read, my family and I have gone through great turmoil gaining access to and controlling spending after both parents became incapacitated. To date, if there is a living will in place for my parents, I do not know about it. What we did get, however, was a beautifully written Power of Attorney.

Since our find, more physicians, lawyers, and care associates have commented on the thoroughness of this particular POA. While I will omit certain obvious names and/or instructions, a copy of it will be provided at the end of this book to offer guidance. Again, the entire purpose of **Operation Caregivers: #LifewithDementia** is to help.

In our parents' individual POA, the specifics come in sections six and seven.

6. SUCCESSOR ATTORNEY-IN-FACT—In the event my wife, Karen W. Powe, is unable or unwilling to serve or continue to serve as my attorney-in-fact, I do hereby make, constitute and appoint my daughter, Alexandra Powe-Allred, an individual residing at ____, as my true and lawful attorney-in-fact with full power and authority as herein before granted.

7. CONTINGENCY—The authority of my wife, Karen W. Powe, and/or my daughter, Alexandra Powe-Allred, as attorney-in-fact to act pursuant to this CONTINGENT DURABLE GENERAL POWER OF ATTORNEY is contingent upon a written determination by a physician then attending me that I am emotionally, physically, or mentally unable or unwilling to properly attend to my affairs or upon the fact that because of my location or physical status I am unable or unwilling to properly attend to my affairs.

Out of more than fourteen in the entire document, those two relatively short directives prove to be the single most important aspect of my parents' POA.

In my mother's paperwork, everything reads the same except in section six, where her directive is, *In the event my husband, Marc B. Powe, is…*and section seven, with the explanation of, *the authority of my husband, Marc B. Powe, and/or my daughter…*

There is no doubt, given of the nature of Daddy's profession, his POA had to be clearly stated in such a manner that Mom and I could move forward in a legal manner should he be kidnapped, held hostage, simply disappear, or be rendered incapacitated. But no matter how thorough he and his lawyer were, detailing what was to be done with receipts, stocks, bonds, debts, bank accounts, real estate, personal property, insurance, tax returns, retirement funds and employee benefits, lending, and more (oh, there is *so* much more), there was never a plan put in action to ensure I was actually made aware of this amazing POA.

It was only when Michelle plowed through piles and files and folders in old office boxes that she happened upon the name of the law firm in Virginia that had helped our father.

A legal plan is a like a chain. It is only as strong as its weakest link. Make sure your appointed POA knows about your legal documents and any legal representation you may have.

What's Your Healthcare Plan?

I've said it before, and I'll say it again—no one ever plans on doing a header on the kitchen floor. No one ever plans on getting dementia.

The questions to ask yourself are *do you have health insurance? Long-term care? Does your doctor understand your long-term medical plans? Do family members know what medications you take or what your medical history looks like? Would they know who to call? Does your Power of Attorney or will stipulate what should be done in the event of a medical or life crisis?* Because I had no knowledge of the POA when everything happened, and because Michelle and I knew so little about their insurance policies, our hunt-and-peck routine took even longer after our parents moved during their own medical crisis. We had no idea.

If we'd only known. Then again, if *if* and *buts* were candy and nuts, we'd have had a fine time.

Admit it. How many times have you seen those commercials for life insurance and rolled your eyes as two or three solemn-looking actors stand around and one says, "I can't believe that Don/Bob/Jim/Joe is gone."

Cue the second actor. "And poor Carol/Jan/Nancy/Mary. She has no way to cover all the medical costs, let along the funeral!"

Now imagine this scene: Michelle and me sitting in our parents' overstuffed, teetering on dangerous, chaotic garage, which is so filled to the brim it would have left the producers of *Hoarders* and *Intervention* drooling with possible showdowns and suspense scenes. We couldn't find anything, not even hope, but Michelle kept saying, again and again, "I know they have some kind of life insurance. I've seen *something*. I know they have something."

They did have something, but it took several hard months and some unfair harassment of New York Life before we discovered what, exactly, they had.

New York Life, in very good faith, honored our parents' requests. Not knowing what those

requests were, however, Michelle and I believed New York Life was holding out on us. It never

occurred to us that our parents, specifically our mother, would dictate their plans not kick in until

one hundred and eighty days after being admitted into memory care, rather than the standard

ninety days.

In Part I of our story, I shared how near crippling those extra ninety days were as we worked

multiple jobs trying to cover Daddy's massive expenses.

Two points need to be made here:

1.   Long-term life insurance should not be looked upon as an unnecessary purchase.

The goal here is exactly as the term describes: health care for the long term. Mom grew

increasingly suspicious of everyone and everything and, at some point, decided she no

longer trusted New York Life. Oh, the irony. She insisted that they revise the plan to

lessen the cost (which on their end was minimal but colossal on ours).

2.   Had a simple file been created, putting the long-term health care policy in the

hands of the POA, we could and would have better understood our situation and been

prepared for it.

Do your due diligence to find the right long-term health insurance company for you and your

family. Make sure that your POA and other family members know your insurance representative

and how to gain information concerning your policy when needed.

Long-Term Medical Plans: Your Doctor, Your Family, and You

You'll recall, in Part I, I also shared a story about Michelle's knowledge about our father's medical history. It was, without exaggeration, life-saving. This said, only sparse details were given about the HIPAA incident.

It is time to share.

One of the most common things family members say about losing a loved one to Alzheimer's or dementia is the feeling of guilt they had for allowing too much time to pass before intervening. They knew *something* was going on.

There's that word: *something*.

There is always *something* with those who are diagnosed (or not yet diagnosed) with Alzheimer's. The trouble starts when you have to figure out what that *something* is. A victim of Alzheimer's also knows *something* is going on, which is why many become more private, very possessive, and incredibly protective of their own personal space and affairs. They can also become secretive and even combative if asked too many questions. The natural inclination is to let them be.

"As long as they aren't burning the house down…"

"As long as they aren't hurting anyone…"

Later, however, family members are left wondering if they could have lessened the progression of the disease, lessened the financial blow, lessened the humiliation or confusion or frustration (for everyone), if had they done *something*.

We knew *something* was going on with both Mom and Daddy, and Michelle tried so hard to get both parents to sign a HIPAA form.

She finally convinced them that she was worried about her own migraines and neck issues and wanted them, her parents, to be able to gain access to her medical file should anything happen. Initially, Mom bought it and signed off.

But afterward, when the doctor's office called and Mom discovered Michelle had access to *their* medical information, she became very angry and accused Michelle of meddling, invading, snooping.

Ironically, it was just two months later that Mom and I sat in the doctor's office, while Daddy was physically restrained in a hospital bed and Mom couldn't recall what month we were in or what year it was, that I gained Medical Power of Attorney the hard way. The as-yet-undiscovered and well-written document from the Virginia law office gave me those rights, but none of the folks who needed to, including me, knew that at the time. If we had, things would have been so much easier.

Case in point, January 12th, Daddy's arrival at the hospital as a John Doe. Mom was completely and utterly clueless about her husband's medical conditions as was I. Because, and only because, Michelle began making private notations of Daddy's medications and, during the move, found his Virginia medical records was someone able to answer the hospital's questions.

You cannot rely on having a Michelle in your life.

Remember that file we talked about creating that includes your POA and insurance information? It should also contain a medical history and complete list of medications.

What Does Your Team Roster Look Like?

Our father was the ultimate team player. That is, until dementia entered our lives. Had he been in the right frame of mind, I believe he would have instructed me what and where and how things were. But the most remarkable thing happened as Alzheimer's began fogging Mom's mind. Daddy's natural inclination was to protect her, circle the wagons, and keep whatever was happening a secret. Then, somewhere along the line, dementia got him. Even more remarkable, Mom could no longer drive, pump gas, go grocery shopping, much less remember how to operate a phone, yet she began covering for her husband as well.

By the time they moved closer to their daughters, Mom and Daddy were deep in the throes of a daily game called, "We can't find Mom's purse. Have you seen it?"

I'm not kidding. It was every stinking day.

Daddy drove, ran errands, got online, paid bill, met with doctors, and made new friends, yet he was also playing the daily "have you seen Mom's purse" game. Instead of asking for help or verbalizing his concerns about his wife's health to us—to *anyone*—he remained mute.

At last, our father reached his own point of no return. His dementia had him unable to see that Mom could not take care of herself. His dementia had him unable to see that he could not take care of his own self.

No one ever plans on face-planting in his own kitchen.

No one ever plans of losing his mind to dementia.

You *can* plan to create your own team.

Why You Need a Team

Tackling Mom and Daddy's financial issues was more than daunting. It was, in the words of one creditor agent, "Unbelievable!" Due to Daddy setting up so many online/automatic payments, paying for things that were clearly a scam, and since I did not yet have a way to stop the financial bleeding, the initial loss was significant.

$29.95 here

$5.89 there

$60.00 here

$32.00 there

All of which added up.

Proving who I was to American Express and VISA, getting Direct TV, various doctors, including the VA, to recognize who I was, and making Publishers Clearing House and a number of charities stop taking money seemed like an endless loop of calls and exhaustive threats each and every day. For the longest time, J C Penny's refused to recognize that our mom—unable to turn her computer on, much less navigate the Internet—could not have possibly hopped online and ordered herself a $900 couch. They have since turned us over to a collection agency, refusing to respond to any of my now five letters addressing Mom's diminished capacity and residency in a memory-care facility upon the date that the couch was purchased.

The only way to manage it all was simple—I had to take time off from work.

But what if I didn't have that luxury?

When you choose your Power of Attorney and/or executor of your will, will this person be able to take an extended period of time away from work, without pay, to handle your affairs?

What you do now, setting things up, and the order of your affairs will greatly impact those you leave behind.

When USAA recognized me fairly quickly (thank you, USAA), and American Express allowed me online access (thank you, American Express), and Wells Fargo helped me establish a new account that coincided with my parents so I could pay bills (thank you, Wells Fargo), I began seeing light at the end of the tunnel. I thought, briefly, maybe, just maybe, I could handle it after all.

When that check to the previous care facility bounced, I panicked.

Thinking it was the only way to keep things afloat, I tried to sell some of my father's stocks to save the house and their credit. In my anxiety over bills and auto withdrawals and, mostly, our parents' plummeting health, I was Chicken Little gone wild. Not only was the sky falling but we also had no money. I was having recurring dreams (or nightmares) where my father was talking to me, but I couldn't understand what he was saying. In one particularly horrid dream, one which I still can't bring myself to relay all the gruesome details, Daddy died on the side of a creek bed, and I just decided to leave him there because, in my dream-state mind, it was easier than the whole process of retrieving his body and taking it somewhere. All I could focus on was being entrusted to take care of things, and it didn't feel like I was doing that at all.

That was when Uncle Stephen stepped in.

Initially, I resisted. Then, my Aunt Diana, in that gentle manner that she has, sent me a note urging me to let Uncle Stephen take the reins of our parents' finances. Even Michelle and Robb urged that I do so, but my ego was in the way. If I let Uncle Stephen take over, hadn't I officially failed my parents? They made me the Power of Attorney and eventual executor of their wills, after all. If I stepped down from this position, in my parents' time of greatest need, wasn't that just too pathetic? They trusted me. Then entrusted me.

It should be mentioned, however, that putting me in charge of their finances should have been a sure sign to the outside world that my dad had onset dementia.

What was he thinking? I have dyscalculia. I barely passed Algebra. I can't even take multiple-choice questionnaires. Seriously. *What was he thinking?!*

Uncle Stephen came at me in a way I couldn't deny. He spoke of teamwork, and that really got me. I'm all about teamwork. My writing career is based upon teams and teamwork, working at the gym, training other people, working with groups, and now caring for our parents—it's all about teamwork. Life is about learning how to work with, enjoy, and succeed with teammates. And so, with math-wizard Uncle Stephen as a new teammate, how could I refuse?

With Uncle Stephen and Aunt Diana officially on board, we had a pretty solid team. Many more, however, were yet to come.

It turns out the Colonel did do some planning, after all, in the form of investments and bonds. He did actually have some money tucked away for this most rainy day. And he had teammates!

Finding the Right Teammates

Once upon a time, I would have thought financial advisors were simply smart people who figured a way to sucker other semi-smart and financially secure people out of their money. Why else would you pay someone to manage your money if you're smart enough to figure out the investment game yourself, right?

Then, I met Jessica Ness from CJM Wealth Advisors, Ltd.

Jessica had been with the company just long enough to have met our father before his move to Texas. In fact, like so many other people, she'd noted at their last meeting, in May of 2014, Daddy had reportedly gotten lost on the way and had been "scattered."

It was more validation that the storm now looming in Daddy's brain had been coming on for some time.

But she also knew him before that "none affective" meeting and liked him.

Like Rose Gentile, of New York Life, Jessica kept notes and was able to advise us on Mom and Daddy's money.

Michelle and I were floundering so long by then that accepting a new team felt amazing. Previously, our team consisted of the caregivers. Even then, our first couple of teams really stunk. They were not true advocates of senior care. They weren't teammates.

As a former sports writer and athlete myself, I often use sport metaphors in life and could not and cannot help but see this as a marathon. Initially, Michelle and I were sprinting but tuckered out pretty quickly. Since then, we've learned to settle in for the big, long, ugly run.

Six months into our marathon with our parents, we had our core runners.

Still, we needed more. Trying to increase our father's benefits with Veterans Affairs was time consuming. Selling Mom's car, halting insurance, shutting down accounts, and moving money was so very tedious. Everything was a battle!

As previously mentioned, I initially believed New York Life was an adversary, working against us for better care, until I began talking to representative Rose Gentile and learned that it was my parents who set up the contract with the extended wait time. Still, New York Life recognized the urgency and double dose of bad we had received and helped. (Thank you, New York Life!)

Jeff Johnson, our parents now-retired accountant, stepped out of the shadows to help, never asking for anything in exchange and Uncle Stephen and Jessica Ness joined forces to figure out long-term financial security for our parents. Wells Fargo Bank, despite whatever negative press they were receiving in the media for a scandal, were our absolute saviors!

Michelle and I were taking our first big, deep breaths in a long time.

As of this writing, we still have some battles to fight. There are still corporations and companies we struggle with, but we will prevail.

Look, Corporate America…we're whirling! We're whirling!

Michelle and I stopped focusing on the obstacles and embraced the team players who were all in. And yeah, this includes all the cheerleaders and well-wishers because, believe you me, they mean *a lot*. But our absolute biggest takeaway is Mom and Daddy are on the team, too. Team Marc-and-Karen isn't just a name. They may not be running the actual steps, but they are most definitely on the team and in the race. We remind ourselves and others that it is essential not to talk about Mom and Daddy in front of Mom and Daddy. Instead, we include them in each conversation, whether they can participate or not.

Chapter Nineteen

FACEBOOK: *September 2017*

> *Mom and I sat on the chairs in the front lobby and watched Ms. Sylvia walk around and around.*
> *Each time she came by, she smiled and said, "Hi, darlin'! Love you."*
> *And I would reply, "Hi! Love you, too!" while Mom scowled at me.*
> *Mom: All she does is walk around and around talking to everyone.*
> *Alex: I know. She's really sweet.*
> *Mom: Who?*
> *Alex: Sylvia.*
> *Mom: Who is Sylvia?*
> *Alex: She…just wait.*
> *[We spoke of other things until Ms. Sylvia came around again.]*
> *Sylvia: Hi, darlin'! How you doing?*
> *Alex: I'm good, Ms. Sylvia. How are you?*
> *Sylvia: I'm good, thank you. Love you.*
> *Alex: Love you, too. [We watch her go] That's Sylvia.*
> *Mom: What about her?*
> *Alex: Nuthin'*
> *Moments later…*
> *Sylvia: Hi, darlin'! Love you.*
> *Alex: Hi!*
> *Mom: Don't talk to her. All she does is walk in circles, talking to everyone.*
> *Alex: Mom, we're all walking in circles right now.*

Whether a person diagnosed with Alzheimer's or dementia should remain at home is a threefold decision. It comes down to *personal*, *financial*, and *medical*.

Because of the very nature of dementia (including Alzheimer's), there is no easy answer. Most of us hope to keep our loved one in his/her own house for as long as possible. That is their home, after all. They are comfortable there. They know where everything is and, until recently, they handled everything just fine.

Ten Things You Should Know About Dementia

1.   **There are over 100 forms of dementia** – Alzheimer's is the most common and accounts for an estimated 50-70 percent of all diagnoses.

2.   **Singling out symptoms** – There is no one single symptom to help diagnose the disease, which is another reason why it goes undiagnosed for so long.

3.   **What are the needs** – Each case and degree of dementia is different, making it more difficult for family to decide how much care is needed. Can they remain living at home? Independently? Or must they go into immediate care to head off any potential dangers?

4.   **More women are affected than men** – According to the Alzheimer's Association, almost two-thirds of Americans with Alzheimer's are women. African-Americans are almost twice as likely to have Alzheimer's or other form of dementia as whites. And in the United Kingdom, 61 percent of dementia patients are women, as opposed to men at 39 percent.[12]

5.   **Dementia is <u>not</u> an "old person's" disease** – Historically, dementia and Alzheimer's have been thought of as only affecting older people and just another reason why it's neglected and marginalized in terms of research and finding a cure. Today, according to the World Health Organization, there are over 47 million people living with dementia with 9.9 million new cases each year. The term "early onset" is becoming more common as more people between the ages of 30 and 65 years old are diagnosed with dementia.

6.   **The age game** – Dementia is not a natural part of aging.

7.   **Health issues can rear dementia's ugly head** – Heart disease raises the risks of a dementia diagnosis. Yet another reason to care for the whole body. Those who suffer from high blood pressure, high cholesterol, diabetes, poor diet, and are otherwise non-active can be at additional risk.

8.   **Sense of smell/taste** – According to the National Institutes of Health, loss of smell and taste have been linked to early signs of Alzheimer's.

9.   **Long-term damage to health** – For caregivers for those living with dementia and Alzheimer's, depression, emotional, and financial stress are a very serious and real issue. It is recommended that caregivers have a social and therapeutic network in place to reduce the risks of psychological and physical illness as well as loss of wages.

---

[12] Dementia Consortium. http://www.dementiaconsortium.org/dementia-facts/

10.   **Independence and dementia** – People with dementia can live independently and remain active for some time after the diagnosis.

Let's talk about #3 and #10 right away.

The diagnosis of dementia is frightening. All too often a family will react strongly to the diagnosis in one of two ways—an over- or under-reaction.

The Overreaction

A loved one diagnosed with dementia or Alzheimer's is immediately put into memory care, whereas this same person could have very successfully continued to live at home with a live-in or visiting caregiver.

This is a hard call.

Do you allow them to live at home and wait for something bad to happen?

There are also many stories of people forced into a memory-care facility in which they are now living with residents who are far more cognitively impaired. This is devastating to a person not yet ready to be in such a place.

Talk to your physician. Ask for an assessment of basic everyday living skills, and talk to different home health agencies who may also assess your loved one.

Many home-health agencies can and will work with your insurance.

Note: Medicare does not cover home health unless this includes skilled nursing care or other physical therapy, occupational therapy, or speech-language pathology services from an accepted home-health agency.

If your loved one needs and/or can obtain assistance, could s/he still live at home?

As described earlier, our situation resolved itself. Michelle lived with our mother until she reached the point that she was waking in the middle of the night, opening the front door, and allowing the dogs to run loose. She capable of operating anything electrical and couldn't understand why she shouldn't operate such things, including the garbage disposal. When she could no longer comprehended a garbage disposal is not turned off by sticking a hand into it, we knew.

By the time we moved her into memory care with our father, she could no longer dress herself or take a shower. She couldn't prepare food for herself and didn't understand how a microwave, much less a stovetop, worked.

The Under-Reaction

People who have been diagnosed with dementia can continue to work, live independently and have a fulfilling social life for an extended period following a diagnosis. Because of this and because symptoms can many times come on rather slowly, family can also be slow to react.

The key to living independently is for a loved one to be able to live safely.

Two of the most common reasons for an under-reaction?

Anosognosia and denial.

What is Anosognosia?

It is *not* denial. It is an unawareness of any kind of impairment.

It is estimated that upward of 81 percent of those with Alzheimer's do not even know they have dementia or any other life-threatening medical issue. It is quite common for them and their family members to put off forgetfulness, confusion, even multiple "clumsy" accidents off to old age.

What is Denial?

Denial is, quite simply, the refusal to accept or acknowledge something; an event, a situation, a claim or a remark. Denial of Alzheimer's and dementia, of course, can not only be dangerous but can bring about disaster, financial ruin, strained relationships, and expedite physical and emotional health for both the patient but also caregivers.

Ten Ways to Identify Denial and/or Anosognosia Amidst Dementia
(For Family/Caregivers)

1.   **Silly ol' senility vs. dementia** – Your grandmother or mother can never find her purse. Your father or uncle is always getting lost. No one knows where the car keys are, and they seem to be keeping odd hours. This is not just normal aging but potential signs of something much bigger on the horizon.

2.   **Accidents** – It's a stumble here, a bruised hip there. When you ask how a bump or scrape happened, your loved one has no idea. These can be precursors of far greater accidents in the coming days and years. Ignoring multiple, seemingly little, accidents can be dangerous. Tripping can lead to broken bones, dislocations, and hospitalization, but there are other kinds of accidents as well. Water left running or the stove left on can lead to even greater accidents. Food poisoning is also an issue among those afflicted with dementia, especially if they lose the sense of smell and taste. They may not know when they are eating something spoiled.

3.   **Avoidance** – Without realizing it, you may have already recognized signs of dementia but have not yet, and do not want to, put a name to it. Instead, you avoid visiting. It is painful to watch your parent or spouse or grandparent fight to find words. It is difficult to watch an otherwise intelligent and funny person struggle with everyday activities. It's much easier to simply not see them.

4.   **Negligent medicating** – You know your loved one needs specific medications and you helpfully lay them all out for him/her to take or, even better, present a weekly pill dispenser, hoping this will keep your loved one on track. But the harsh reality is, all or none of the pills might be consumed. They could end up lost, misplaced, thrown away, or all consumed at once. This is a dangerous game to play with someone who exhibiting odd or unusual behavior. Denial with medication can most certainly bring out dangerous results.

5.   **Overindulging** – You know something is wrong but…what? Rather than getting to the root of the problem, you simply present them with gifts, goodies, or surprises to make them happy. Rather than question the number of packages that appear at the front door day after day, where the medication has gone, why the phone is never answered, you present gifts and goodies.

6.   **Rift among family** – Not everyone is on the same page. Suddenly, you have cousins or old family friends questioning you about your loved one's current situation. It may feel like a personal attack. Inquiries from neighbors may feel intrusive. Or, the family may be divided on

what is really wrong with dad. The fact that questions are being asked about changes in behavior or living situations is a red flag.

7.   **The Money Tree** – Managing money is one of the first skills that eludes a person with dementia. Because of the compulsivity link to dementia, the lack of inhibition and restrains, people with dementia will suddenly spend money as though they have a money tree in their backyard. Like our father, some will become very charitable, wanting to help others and change the world. Others will become unusually excited about "deals" on TV, wanting to order every great product they see. Ignoring these behaviors could cost more than what you see leaving the bank account as they open themselves up to fraud and scams, forgetting to pay bills and losing their credit card information. Remember that dementia is a progressive disease and these behaviors will only worsen.

8.   **Your own health** – Until this time, you have been trying to do it all. According to the Caregiver Family Alliance, most (family) caregivers are ill-prepared for the role of caregiver. In fact, the statistics among family caregivers for depression, anxiety, emotional and physical distress, overall health and life expectancy are staggering.[13]

Beyond the physical care of your loved one, there are many legal, financial, medical and personal issues to be taken care of. As dementia moves into your lives, it is imperative that you are able and willing to take care of these issues for your loved one. Learning to delegate for your health and that of your entire family must be considered.

9.   **The Great Communicator** – Part of your denial might be this: You are embarrassed. Suddenly, your spouse or parent is blurting out inappropriate things and so, in protection of your loved one, you constantly make excuses. Time and again, we would see this with our own parents. Before our father's dementia took hold, he was making one excuse after another for our mother and why it was she could not attend a wedding, a party, a social function in the neighborhood. In hopes of protecting her, he allowed for her to hide from the world. In the end, this only made things worse for Mom, made her more reclusive and afraid, but it also made things far more difficult for family and friends, who felt blindsided and frustrated.

10.   **Legal standing** – It is here that denial is most costly. With dementia, you never know when the next accident or disaster is coming. Being caught unprepared could cost thousands of dollars but also the proper care your loved one needs. You have noted that something is wrong

---

[13] https://www.caregiver.org/caregiver-health

with your spouse, parent, or sibling, but you don't want to take any kind of action for fear of appearing intrusive, disrespectful, or even greedy. The reality is, you need financial and medical power of attorney. You need to be able to give medical directive, see health records, and speak to doctors. You will need to be able to shut down accounts, stop automatic payments, speak to bankers, and control money for the care of your loved one.

How to Get Power of Attorney

The entire purpose of *Operation Caregivers: #LifewithDementia* is to prevent this very discussion.

It is our hope that a Power of Attorney has already been named for you and your loved ones. However, we know better. For this reason, a list of helpful suggestions as to how to obtain this legal standing has been provided but it is not foolproof. Every dementia patient is different. Part of the disease (and its progression) is about altered reality, growing paranoia, and fear. Confusion and altered reality can make a loved one defiant, refusing any and all help.

For these reasons, you may have to move carefully, always remembering how upsetting this is to your loved one.

Ten Ways You May Obtain Power of Attorney/Legal Guardianship

1. **Capacity assessment** – Make an appointment with your loved one's primary physician or general practitioner. In making this appointment, make it clear that you hope to be in attendance and explain to the nurse what has been going on with your loved one. This doesn't mean you will be allowed into the assessment and, in fact, you may be excluded from sitting in, depending upon the state of dementia and mood. Be prepared.

2. **HIPAA documentation** – If you are able to gain access to HIPAA, this can be the first step in getting medical power of attorney. Easier said than done, however, if your loved one refuses to sign the paperwork. This is a trust issue for your loved one and they must be in agreement to share their medical information with you with the doctor.

3. **Support groups** – If met with serious resistance from a person who has dementia from gaining medical/financial POA, include support groups. Bring the capacity assessment to a meeting you have established between the support group, you and your loved one. Perhaps you can even leave the room and allow for an elderly and/or dementia representative to speak to your family member or friend who is suffering (even unknowingly) from the disease.

4.   **Proven and professional resources** – a number of organization, such as the Alzheimer's Association, have trained representative who can counsel you on how to move forward with or without your loved one. *See **Additional Resources** for organizations.

5.   **Include family** – Theft and fraud against the elderly is a rising crime, not only in the United States but also across the globe. In fact, a study in the U.K. found that of the financial abusers against the elderly, 53 percent of the theft, fraud and deception was committed by the victim's middle-aged children.[14] For this reason, keeping the family informed is imperative. A 'full disclosure' attitude will not only impress the courts and/or lawyers, it will strengthen the family, possibly prevent another family member from accusing you of taking advantage of the situation but, frankly, will help you resist any temptation from abusing your power.

6.   **Include friends** – All too often, the natural inclination is to keep this a secret. Alzheimer's and dementia are a global affair. It affects us all. Your husband or wife's friends, those closest to your parents or grandparents may be your best ally in this fight against dementia. Include them in what is happening and arrange for a meeting among friends. Let them share with your loved one how they have created a wellness and welfare plan for their own future. Then have a few of those friends suggest including you in on their next discussion and have a strategy as to how to create a power of attorney for you. Your local support and/or Alzheimer's organizations can be very helpful here.

7.   **Start documenting now** – Begin documenting everything. Create a timeline of when you noticed your loved one's difficulty in properly caring for him/herself; write down any instances of getting lost, fender-bender car accidents (no matter how seemingly minor); financial confusion or difficulties, unexplained medical or legal issues. Note change in behavior and relations with friends, family, and neighbors.

8.   **Legal help** – Contact your local Eldercare locator at (800) 677-1116 or visit www.eldercare.gov for free legal resources or contact the National Academy of Elder Law Attorneys to find someone nearest you at www.NAELA.org

9.   **Living or Last Will** – The discovery of a living or last will can be used as a type of "advance directive" in the legal system. If you are named as executor, this could help prove that

---

[14] Woman, S., "Elderly Most At Risk of Theft By Own Children," The Telegraph. January 30, 2007. http://www.telegraph.co.uk/news/uknews/1540982/Elderly-most-at-risk-of-theft-by-own-children.html

your loved one does have faith in you to take care of him or her and may be used to give you legal standing to gain guardianship. Again, legal advice and guidance is advised.

10.   **Your loved one** – Dementia and Alzheimer's is a surprising disease. There can be times during the day when your loved one is more lucid and amenable. Do not accuse a person living with dementia of forgetting or losing something as a way of convincing them to give you power of attorney. Rather, use the example of a friend or someone in the news as a reason why you hope to have the family come together and everyone, young and old, create a long-term wellness and welfare plan. If the timing is right, you might be able to obtain a power of attorney status directly from your loved one.

For us, it was not until our father's fall that Mom gave up the "we'll be just fine without you" claims. For the first time, she was truly scared. For what we now know to be over a decade, her protector was no longer by her side, making up excuses for her as to why she could not attend a party or find her purse. Each day, however vulnerable she was, she would threaten to call a lawyer on us, she would claim that she was going to find the GPS and start driving again (we hid the keys), she said she would call the police and did. But we also found times where she wanted and needed us and was open to discussions about her future. Here, we knew, we had to be very cautious. Any perceived threat of taking away her independence, her way of living, her say in a medical or legal matter (though in the moments that most mattered, she had none to offer), would enrage her.

Before we found our parents' lawyer in Virginia, before we thought we had any legal position at all, we were able to convince Mom, for the sake of proper medical treatment for our father, to meet with a lawyer and give us medical power of attorney.

Our Personal Top Ten Ways of Obtaining POA for Mom

1.   **Capacity assessment** – Using Mom's primary physician, who she had decided she did not trust, as she had stopped trusting anyone who might give her unwanted advice, we were able to do an assessment on Mom to determine her current condition.

2.   **HIPAA** – While in the hospital, visiting Daddy, we were able to get Mom to sign a HIPAA form, for Daddy's sake. This way, we told her, we were all able to talk about Daddy's medical condition. Mercifully, this was actually true.

3.   **Include family** – We made sure that our aunts and uncles were all aware of what was happening, but also included extended family members and friends of our parents. This was done to gather more medical and/or counseling advice but also a way to ensure a 'full disclosure' to all as to what was happening and what we were trying to accomplish with Mom.

4.   **Include friends** – I began writing/e-mailing friends of the family to enlist help for Mom. Of all the steps, this was the least helpful in that Mom had already become so withdrawn from everyone that she no longer felt any deep connection but for Ms. Pat. I was able to remind her again and again how brilliantly Ms. Pat had planned her own power of attorney, will, living and funeral arrangements. However, on a personal note, including friends was most helpful to Michelle and I as we began to hear stories we never knew before (examples of times Mom and/or Daddy appeared "out of it") and were able to create more of a timeline.

5.   **Start documenting now** – I created a timeline of Mom's reclusive and hoarding behaviors, events in which she forgot smaller things (how to eat pizza) and bigger things (forgetting that Daddy had had a heart monitor). My timeline coincided with our doctor on date, time and place when Mom could not recall what day, month, or even year we were living in.

6.   **Financial leverage** – Once again, I used my own father as leverage in getting Mom to accept that we needed legal help to access accounts, medical records and financial statement to assure Daddy's welfare. In doing this, I had asked Mom several questions about bank statements and payments that I knew she would not be able to answer. When she could not, I appeared alarmed and exclaimed, "We need to get help! And fast!" This worked. Together, we went to the bank so she could see we were a team.

7.   **Property leverage** – Similar to the banking situation, I asked questions about the house in regards to mortgage payments and equity in the home. When Mom could not answer (and knew that Daddy could not answer for her), she agreed to talk to someone about her home.

8.   **Legal help** – After calling around to a few lawyers, a great one was recommended to help with our unique situation. I made sure to write up a more detailed account of what was going on and forward it ahead so that the team would be fully apprised of Mom's state of mind and medical condition. We received great counsel both with and without Mom.

9.   **Exploration** – In our quest to find something, anything to help gain greater legal footing, Michelle found a letter from a lawyer in Virginia who sounded like he had done some kind of legal work for Mom and Daddy. I called and discovered there was, in fact, a power of attorney. Hallelujah! In truth, we were just looking for something akin to a will and had no idea such a great POA even existed. Leave nothing to chance and go through every letter and file your family member may have that can assist you in court. Reminder: Mom's "filing system" was insane. Don't assume that a POA or insurance information will be in a file marked *POA* or *Insurance*. The POA could be in a sewing kit!

10.   **Mom** – There were days when she was quite ugly about things. We learned when to walk away, when to come back in for a second or third round. But it always had to be Mom's idea. In the end, going to see a lawyer, having an appointment with the doctor, talking to bank managers and mortgage brokers had to be Mom's idea. At all times, we tried to keep Mom empowered in her own affairs—even if we were pulling all the strings.

Again, we had no knowledge of an existing POA set up by a law firm in another state. My response was launching into my own proactive procurement of POA for our mother. Because every situation is so different—in our case, our mother resisted us at almost every turn--we're sharing this information only as a helpful guide.

As you gain control over the medical and legal aspects of caregiving and your loved one, a major decision regarding living must be made. So often, the decision is made for a family due to certain situations. This chapter opened with the statement that there are three major dictators to how your loved one can/will be cared for in regards to homecare vs. facility care:

- ❖ Personal
- ❖ Financial

❖ Medical

Whether this is a personal choice or something that must be done for financial or medical reasons, choosing at-home care can be both gratifying and challenging.

At-home (or in-home) care is a massive decision that cannot possibly be fit into a Top Ten advice column. There are many choices and services that go with at-home care, from companion and personal care services to help with housekeeping, shopping and meal preparation. Skilled nurses are also available to help with physical therapy, wound care, and medication.

Your insurance coverage will most likely hinge of what kind of care is available to your loved one.

Before considering at-home care, reach out to your team.

Ten People or Organizations to Speak with Before Considering At-Home Care

1.   **Medical insurance** – Learn what is covered with home health care, what is expected of you (as caregiver), and what kind of compensation you can expect.

2.   **Long-term/Life insurance** – Speak to a representative of the life insurance policy your loved one may hold to determine if the at-home care you have selected qualifies for the kind of care specified in the policy. Typically, these policies are very specific about how and where care is given to the policyholder.

3.   **Primary physician** – Speak to your doctor about this decision and what is best for your family. Be prepared to hear what a trained professional may think about this decision. Just because you think this is a good idea or your only recourse, your doctor may know better. Be open to other idea on how best to care for your loved one. At one point, Michelle suggested she become a full-time caregiver for Mom, but many of us nixed this idea immediately. Not only was Mom far beyond Michelle's abilities, but also Michelle, given to reclusive behavior and depression, would have been emotionally destroyed in this process.

4.   **Family** – Be sure to include family in this big decision. Because this is such a big decision, you will need other family to fall on when you are ill, must travel, want to get away for a vacation, or just need to go to the grocery store.

5.   **Alzheimer's and dementia support groups** – These organizations have and provide excellent resources for at-home services but can also counsel you in coping with this new 'round the clock' job. Joining a support group is a great (and healthy) way to stay abreast of new information regarding home health, insurance, better care, support systems and counseling for you.

6.   **Talk to other at-home care family members** – using an Alzheimer's group and/or at-home chat sites, find a few people in a similar situation and inquire about the day-to-day experiences of at-home care. Don't just talk to the professionals, but ask family members what it is like to care for a loved one at home.

7.   **Home health services** – Whether you want to use a home health service or not, it would be wise to speak to a representative from four or five different companies to list and compare the kind of services that are available. They can also determine how your medical insurance coverage can be best utilized in caring for your loved one. You may learn a few things just from a simple interview process.

8.   **Consider adult day centers** – Better yet, consider visiting the day center with your loved one to see if s/he qualifies to attend. These centers offer structure and familiarity, while also offering a safe haven while you are away. Most offer music, art therapy, game time, even field trips.

9.   **Legal support** – Before making this decision, speak to a lawyer about home health and homeowner's insurance. Assuming you have power of attorney, you want to make sure you are honoring the POA and, if there is a living will, any documents that may have been created by your loved one. Because elder fraud is so prevalent, you want to be sure you are doing everything properly in the eyes of the law, your doctor's and family in caring for your loved one.

10.   **Neighbors** – Your first inclination may be to think, 'this isn't any of their business.' Think again. While their opinion should not matter in how you care for your loved one, you do want your neighbors aware of your intentions to keep your loved one at home for care. Wandering, calling police and the fire department, calling out for help and/or yelling are common issues with those living with dementia. By talking to neighbors about your intentions you are both informing them of what could potentially occur, asking them for an extra bit of understanding.

Finally, before taking on such a life-changing job, consider this wonderful list created by the Family Caregiver Alliance and National Center on Caregiving. This advice is perfect for anyone caring for and loving someone with dementia.

Ten Real-Life Strategies for Dementia Caregiving

1.   **Being reasonable, rational, and logical will just get you into trouble** – When someone is acting in ways that don't make sense, we tend to carefully explain the situation, calling on his or her sense of appropriateness to get compliance. However, the person with dementia doesn't have a "boss" in his brain any longer, so he does not respond to our arguments, no matter how logical. Straightforward, simple sentences about what is going to happen are usually the best.

2.   **People with dementia do not need to be grounded in reality** – When someone has memory loss, he often forgets important things, e.g., that his mother is deceased. When we remind him of this loss, we remind him about the pain of that loss also. When someone wants to go home, reassuring him that he is at home often leads to an argument. Redirecting and asking someone to tell you about the person he has asked about or about his home is a better way to calm a person with dementia.

3.   **You cannot be a perfect caregiver** – Just as there is no such thing as a perfect parent, there is no such thing as a perfect caregiver. You have the right to the full range of human emotions, and sometimes you are going to be impatient or frustrated. Learning to forgive your loved one as well as yourself is essential in the caregiving journey.

4.   **Therapeutic lying reduces stress** – We tend to be meticulously honest with people. However, when someone has dementia, honesty can lead to distress both for us and the one we are caring for. Does it really matter that your loved one thinks she is the volunteer at the day care center? Is it okay to tell your loved one that the two of you are going out to lunch and then "coincidentally" stop by the doctor's office on the way home to pick something up as a way to get her to the doctor?

5.   **Making agreements don't work** – If you ask your loved one to not do something ever again, or to remember to do something, it will soon be forgotten. For people in early stage dementia, leaving notes as reminders can sometimes help, but as the disease progresses, this will not work. Taking action, rearranging the environment, rather than talking and discussing, is usually a more successful approach. For example, getting a teakettle with an automatic "off" switch is better than warning someone of the dangers of leaving the stove on.

6.   **Doctors often need to be educated by you** – Telling the doctor what you see at home is important. The doctor can't tell during an examination that your loved one has been up all night

pacing. Sometimes doctors need to deal with therapeutic lying as well (e.g., telling the patient that an antidepressant is for memory rather than depression).

7.   **You can't do it all** – When people offer to help, the answer should always be a resounding *yes*. It's okay. Have a list of things people can do to help you, whether it is bringing a meal, picking up a prescription, helping trim the roses, or staying with your loved one while you run an errand. This will reinforce offers of help. It is harder to ask for help than to accept it when it is offered, so don't wait until you "really need it" to get support.

8.   **It is easy to both overestimate and underestimate what your loved one can do** – It is often easier to do something for our loved ones than to let them do it for themselves. However, if we do it for them, they will lose the ability to be independent in that skill. On the other hand, if we insist individuals do something for themselves and they get frustrated, we just make our loved one's agitated and probably haven't increased their abilities to perform tasks. Not only is it a constant juggle to find the balance, but be aware that the balance may shift from day to day.

9.   **Tell, don't ask** – Asking, "What would you like for dinner?" may have been a perfectly normal question at another time. But now we are asking our loved one to come up with an answer when he or she might not have the words for what they want, might not be hungry, and even if they answer, might not want the food when it is served after all. Saying "We are going to eat now" encourages the person to eat and doesn't put them in the dilemma of having failed to respond.

10.   **It is perfectly normal to question the diagnosis during moments of lucidity** – One of the hardest things to do is to remember that we are responding to a disease, not the person who once was. Everyone with dementia has times when they make perfect sense and can respond appropriately. We often feel like that person has been faking it or that we have been exaggerating the problem when these moments occur. We are not imagining things—they are just having one of those moments, to be treasured when they occur.[15]

---

[15] https://www.caregiver.org/ten-real-life-strategies-dementia-caregiving

Ten Things You Need Before Hiring Professional Care

1.   **Home safety** – Screen your applicants thoroughly! Check references, do background checks, ask for certificates. Although there are many reliable and competent caregivers working independently, seniors are prime targets for abuse. You need to take all precautions to ensure that your helper is in good faith. Additionally, secure valuables. This is a safety precaution for everyone.

2.   **Immigration status** – All employers must make sure an employee is eligible to work in the United States and file an I-9 form, which contains instructions on how to verify eligibility.

3.   **Employer Identification Number (EIN)** Household employers do not need a business license, but they do need an EIN, which is not the same as a social security number. You can obtain an EIN by applying online with the IRS. Web site. EINs are provided free of charge and will be used on tax forms you file for your employee.

4.   **Social security and Medicare taxes** – If you pay a household employee cash wages of a specified amount or more in a calendar year ($1,800 or more for 2013, $1,900 or more for 2014), you generally must withhold 6.2% of social security and 1.45% of Medicare taxes from all wages you pay to that employee. Unless you prefer to pay your employee's share of social security and Medicare taxes from your own funds, you should withhold 7.65 percent from each payment of cash wages made.

5.   **Federal income tax withholding** – You are not required to withhold federal income tax from wages you pay to a household employee. However, if your employee asks you to withhold federal income tax and you agree, you will need a completed Form W-4 (Employee's Withholding Allowance Certificate) from your employee.

6.   **Form W-2, wage and tax statement** – You will need to complete form W-2 (Wage and Tax Statement) for each employee. You will also need a W-3 form, which is Transmittal of Wage and Tax Statement, and you'll also have to file Schedule H (household employment tax form) with your own federal tax return each April.

7.   **Federal Unemployment Tax Act (FUTA)** – If you paid wages to household employees totaling more than $1,000 in any calendar quarter during the calendar year or the prior year, you generally must pay federal unemployment tax on the first $7,000 of wages you pay to each household employee. Generally, you can take a credit against your FUTA tax liability for amounts you paid into state unemployment funds. A state that has not repaid money it borrowed

from the federal government to pay unemployment benefits is a "credit reduction state." If you paid wages that are subject to the unemployment compensation laws of a credit reduction state, your FUTA tax credit may be reduced.

8.   **State payroll taxes** – In addition to federal taxes, employers also pay and/or withhold state payroll taxes. These may include employment training tax, state disability insurance, personal income tax, and unemployment taxes.

9.   **Workers' compensation insurance** – Many states, including California, require employers to have workers' compensation insurance, even if they have only one employee. Visit taxes.ca.gov to learn more about the state payroll tax obligations.

10.   **Record keeping** – Keep copies of every time sheet, pay stub, every form you file and proof of all payments from your bank. The IRS suggests keeping records for at least four years after the due date of your tax return or the date you actually paid the taxes, whichever is later.

Alzheimer's Association also recommends that you contract a payroll agency, such as PayChex, NannyChex, or HomeWork Solutions, "considering all that could go wrong when failing to comply with household employer's obligations."[16] You can also use software that allows you to create your own payroll and follow set contracts.

Whether you hire independently or work to find a caregiver/skilled nurse through an agency, you should have set criteria that goes beyond payroll. You'll want and need someone who will care for your loved one regardless of their uncharacteristic and unbecoming, yet typical, behaviors of dementia. Another purpose of this book is to help others avoid as much of the lack of care and training and compassion that we experienced with women who did not understand dementia and should never have entered the caregiving profession.

---

[16] https://www.alz.org/cacentral/documents/Professional_Care_29_-_Hiring_In-Home_Helpers.pdf

Chapter Twenty

Who and What is Caregiver?

That amazing moment when you walk into memory care, come around the corner, and see your mom smiling and dancing with her beautiful caregivers and realize, "She's okay, She's okay!"
Now, the bigger decision. Run or join 'em?

There are two different kinds of caregivers. There is the informal caregiver—the family member, friend of the family, or neighbor, for example, who do what they do out of love and/or necessity, and usually unpaid or may be paid under the table—then, there is the formal caregiver. The formal caregiver is a paid professional care provider, typically working with an agency, a residential or long-term-care facility, daycare, or hospital.

The Informal Caregiver

- ❖ **The care at-home ratio** – An estimated 43.5 million adults in the U.S. provided unpaid care for a loved one in 2016.

- ❖ **At-home care for dementia** – Approximately 15.7 million adult caregivers provided home care for a family member diagnosed with Alzheimer's or dementia.[17]

- ❖ **Gender caregiving** – Women are the majority of caregivers, numbering 60 percent of all care at home.

- ❖ **Caregiver ratio** – Of the caregivers surveyed, eight in 10 responded to only caring for one person who is a relative. In fact, 85 percent of home-care recipients are family.[18]

- ❖ **Informal or formal care** – Fifty-Seven percent of caregivers report that they do not have a choice in performing at-home care. Forty-three percent have no one else to perform the needed care or do not have insurance to pay for professional or formal care. Twelve percent reported feeling pressure or guilt to care for a family member by the recipient of the care, and eight percent felt pressured by other family members to perform the care

[17] Alzheimer's Association. (2015). 2015 Alzheimer's Disease Facts and Figures
[18] AARP Public Policy Institute, 2015 Report: Caregiving in the U.S.
http://www.aarp.org/content/dam/aarp/ppi/2015/caregiving-in-the-united-states-2015-report-revised.pdf

duties.[19] Most middle-class families report that they cannot afford the average cost for skilled or formal care, which averages $18/hour for personal aides and $19/hour home health aides. *Agencies take roughly half of that pay.

❖ **Age** – The average age of the informal caregiver is 49.2 years. 48 percent of those caregivers are between the ages of 18 to 49. Thirty-four percent are over the age of 65.[20]

❖ **Work and caregiving** – Six in 10 caregivers experienced negative impact on work, having to cut back hours, take a leave of absence, or being reprimanded for poor work performance, as a few examples. The higher the need of the care recipient, the more impactful it is on job performance.

❖ **What is time** – Depending on the level of health and needs of the loved one, more time is needed for care. For primary family caregivers caring for a loved one with dementia, an average of nine hours per day is required. One in four caregivers report giving an average of upward to 75 hours a week in home care.[21]

❖ **Present plans** – At-home caregivers report that they need more information in regards to caregiving topics, such as dementia, incontinence, managing their own stress, and even making end-of-life decisions. Eight out of ten (84 percent) feel disconnected from proper medical and caregiving guidance.

❖ **Future plans** – Of the caregiver between the ages of 18 to 49, just 34 percent have made arrangements for long-term care, insurance, Power of Attorney, and medical directives, while those ages 75 and older have. Seventy-eight percent of older caregivers have made future plans. Income coincides with these plans. For those earning $50,000 to $99,999 a year, almost 50 percent have made provisions. As the income drops so, too, does planning for the future.

In 2015, there were more than 14.9 million caregivers providing care for someone living with Alzheimer's or other dementia. These numbers are changing daily as more and more people are being diagnosed with the disease. Eighty percent of elderly receiving assistance living at home

---

[19] AARP and United Health Hospital Fund. (2012). Home Alone: Family Caregivers Providing Complex Chronic Care.]
[20] National Alliance for Caregiving and AARP. (2015). Caregiving in the U.S.]
[21] Fisher, G. G., Franks, M. M., Plassman, B. L., Brown, S. L., Potter, G. G., Llewellyn, D., et al. (2011). Caring for Individuals with Dementia and Cognitive Impairment, not Dementia: Findings from the Aging, Demographics, and Memory Study

rather than a residential or long-term facility. For these reasons, the numbers on just how many caregivers are in the United States alone, as skewed. But we do know that the need for caregivers has skyrocketed.

According to the United States Department of Labor, in a 2014 report of fastest growing occupations (and the need thereof), personal care aides was No.1. In fourth place was home health aides and nursing assistants was listed as number six.[22]

For each position, the Bureau of Labor presented an estimated number to fulfill need at a combined total of 1.3 million new jobs, but PHI, a healthcare organization (formerly known as Paraprofessional Healthcare Institute) believes more are needed. PHI predicted that by the year 2020, "direct-care" will become the largest occupation in the United States.[23]

The Formal (Professional) Caregiver

Depending on where you live, the following information can be gratifying or horrifying. Formal personal and health care aides remain a state-by-state regulatory occupation.

Dog training, as one example, has always been an unregulated profession. Anyone could slap a choke or shock collar on a dog and call him or herself a professional dog trainer. Germany became the first country to make animal training a protected or regulated profession. The United States remains one of many that allows "professionals" to exists state-by-state. Dog lover that I am, there is quite a difference between dog training and working with/caring for someone with

---

[22] United States Department of Labor: Bureau of Labor Statistics.
https://www.bls.gov/news.release/ecopro.t05.htm
[23] Graham, J. "A Shortage of Caregivers," New York Times. February 26, 2014.
https://newoldage.blogs.nytimes.com/2014/02/26/a-shortage-of-caregivers/

dementia. Yet, each state and its requirements of how much training a "professional" must have varies greatly.

In the states of New Jersey and Washington, each requires 75 or more hours of training before a professional can be staffed by a licensed agency and must carry two different home care licenses. Further, in Washington state, a professional must have 85 hours of training before becoming a certified nurse's aide (CAN). However, every other state within the United States only requires EIGHT hours of training to care for our elderly. California requires ten hours.

In Alabama, there are no licensing requirements and no non-medical training hours required.[24] Because this remains a relatively low-skills, low-professional occupation, it does not require much training or education. Thus, many of the "professionals" are anything but.

The irony here is this: This is actually a very HIGH skills job. Great caregivers are incredibly insightful and often know of or are aware of a medical issue before the medical professionals are. The occupation of caregiving is an extremely intense, difficult, demanding job that is complicated by numerous medical issues and demands. The level of knowledge, patience, energy, and professionalism that this occupation requires is astounding. Arguably, this is the single most undervalued, marginalized job in the world and something needs to change.

Author's Note: Caregivers Action Network (CAN) is an excellent non-profit organization dedicated to providing education, peer support, and resources to family caregivers across the country free of charge. Talk to them about how you can improve care in your state. www.caregiveraction.org OR contact your local and state representative to demand better training for increased salary for professional caregivers.

---

[24] https://www.caregiverlist.com/Caregiver-Training-Requirements-By-State.aspx

These caregivers do incredible work and the demand for more grows every day. They bathe, dress, feed and comfort, they care for and cater to those living with disability, senior age, and/or the very debilitating disease of dementia. Whether in private or group homes, assisted living centers, adult day centers, rehabilitative or long-term memory-care facilities, they are caring for our families, for our future.

Hiring a Formal Caregiver

Should you have the means and/or ability to keep your loved one at home, there are some things to consider before hiring (and sustaining) a caregiver.

If you are looking for skilled nursing and/or professional care in the home, there are numerous agencies in your area. Using Alzheimer's Association or other dementia organizations to find excellent resources, or contact Elder Care.

However, should you decide to hire a caregiver directly, there are some things you need to consider. By doing this, you are becoming an employer and must then assume responsibility for all fiscal employment obligations. Alzheimer's Association compiled a great list of what you must consider before hiring a caregiver to remain compliant with federal law:

Ten Things You Should <u>Care</u> About Professional Caregivers

1.   **Understanding of dementia** – Dementia is not the same as senior aging or experiencing memory loss. Dementia is a disease. It is a disorder of the mental process that changes personality, impairs reasoning, and bring about tremendous frustration and confusion for its victim. A caregiver who truly understands that the actions of a person with dementia is not to blame or is not at fault for his or her own actions.

2.   **Understanding family** – Not only does a good caregiver understand her charge but can also empathize with what the family is going through. In fact, a good caregiver will often counsel family members, reminding them, "This isn't your Papa. You know that, right? He can't help himself. He doesn't know what he is doing." And should your loved one do something shocking like undress or become violent, the caregiver will reassure you that this behavior is not unusual and no one is upset or disappointed with your loved one.

3.   **Personal background** – It is helpful when a caregiver knows how you feel because they went through something similar with a family member. Very often, these events of caring for a loved one are what encouraged the caregiver into this profession. Feeling some kind of kinship or connection to the person caring for your loved one can be very empowering. Do not be afraid to ask your caregiver how s/he became a nurse or caregiver.

4.   **Professionalism** – While the caregiver can (you hope) share personal stories with you, this should not include financial woes. One of the top complaints among family members in elder care is this: caregivers hit up families for extra cash with the implication of 'so I can keep taking good care of your loved one.' Their personal problems should not be put on you or your family as this can often feel like emotional warfare.

5.   **Commitment (aka not texting, aka changing diapers)** – Recently, my daughter called me to tell me she found an elderly woman in her apartment complex, 'huffing, puffing, and sweating,' and she asked the woman if she was okay. The woman replied that she needed to get to the pharmacy to get her medication and, that because her caregiver left early, she would have to walk there to get it for herself. Sadly, this is not uncommon for a family to hire a caregiver only to learn, often when it is too late, that the caregiver was privately keeping her own hours for personal time.

Caregivers must understand that theirs is a very demanding job. Each and every day they must be 'up' for whatever challenge comes their way. Declaring that certain unpleasant tasks "isn't my job," or talking on the phone while on the clock is not acceptable. Pay attention to how committed your caregiver truly is.

6.   **Patience** – This is so important as this very quality—patience—is tried each and every hour, if not minute when caring for those with dementia. Caregivers should be able and willing to repeat themselves over and over, each time with equal amount of love and understanding. Facial expression, tone of voice, and general attitude ARE conveyed to those with dementia. While the patient/resident may not understand the words, they can feel how their caregiver feels about them.

7.   **Language barriers** – This is a difficult challenge as a rising number of caregiver do not speak English as a first or primary language. Fair or not, the thicker the accent, the more difficult it could be for your loved one to understand and take directives. If you can't understand your caregiver, imagine how frustrating this might be for your loved one who is already in a heightened state of confusion and agitation. It is imperative that whoever your caregiver is, a sense of calm is always present.

8.   **Taskmaster** – Whether your caregiver is working one-on-one with your loved one or is an employee of a larger facility with a number of charges, it is important that s/he be able to manage many things at the same time. It is important that s/he not get flustered when multiple things are happening. In the end, you want to know that this person will not panic or overreact to something and will be able to help your loved one in a moment of chaos or crisis.

9.   **Schedule-master** – Along with being a taskmaster, you want to have a caregiver who can stick to a schedule for your loved one. Naturally, meal times and dispensing of medication are important, but so are those times when they might go walking, watch TV, go for a ride, and play BINGO. Consistency, especially for those living with dementia, is so important. In keeping with being a schedule-master, the caregiver is reliable and punctual, rarely calling in sick or requesting personal time. Though they may not be able to articulate such things, your loved one will come to depend upon and look for their caregiver. Consistency = Security.

10.   **Education** – As mentioned at the beginning of this section, education is sorely lacking in this industry. Look for that special caregiver who goes beyond what is required to learn about and earn additional certifications regarding dementia, Parkinson's, anxiety disorders, etc. The more knowledge they acquire, the most confident and competent they become.

Ten Things Your Caregiver Should Know about <u>You!</u>

It is equally important that you share in this experience. To be fair, there are things caregivers wish you understood. Compiled is a top ten list from caregivers in long-term facilities.

1.   **Ability to listen** – For the more experienced caregivers who have been providing care for the elderly and/or those with dementia for many years, they can often see or predict a problem before anyone else. Many recognize a UTI (urinary tract infection), dehydration, negative reaction to a medication, or even a change in behavior before anything happens sooner than family or physicians. Because they spend day in/day out with their residents, they have a much keener sense of what is happening. When they talk to you, they need for you to heed their concerns or warnings for the sake of your loved one.

2.   **Supplying what is needed** – Whether your loved one is at home or in a facility, there are certain things that may be needed, such as new clothing, shampoo, a kind of lotion or soap. Because those living with Alzheimer's have very sensitive feet, special socks and slippers are always needed (especially since those with dementia also love to hide said slippers). When caregivers ask for something in particular, it is for a reason and they need you to help them help your loved one.

3.   **Following the plan** – For many caregivers, this is a recurring problem. Caregivers like to bring order to the otherwise chaotic life of a person with dementia. If they share a routine with you, they do so in hopes of you following along to help your loved feel some semblance of structure. Just because it doesn't fit in with your plans for the day doesn't mean this is good for your spouse or parent or grandparent. Please be mindful of their pre-set schedule.

4.   **One at a time, please** – However great the intentions, too many relatives offering too many ideas about how to care for their patient or resident can be incredibly stressful, even harmful to the caregiver and your loved one.

5.   **Taking constructive criticism** – For caregivers, this may be the most difficult task of all—how to instruct the family member for better care.

Example: a family member routinely arriving too close to bedtime or just as medicine is being dispensed, only to rile up the patient, then leaving.

Or, a family member visits, each time bringing a venti mega-mocha Frappuccino for his mother which gives her terrible diarrhea but despite being told, continues the pattern because it makes his mother "happy."

Or, a family member constantly changing things in her loved one's room but the change is upsetting to the loved on.

Are you open to constructive criticism if it is helpful to your loved one? Caregivers are often afraid to speak up on behalf of their patient or resident for fear of angering or upsetting the family member. Let them know you want to help and are open to suggestions for the sake of your loved one.

6.   **Accessibility** – Unlike the formal at-home caregiver, often the caregiver who works in a residential or long-term facility rarely sees the family members. *Where are you?* According to a review in the National Institute of Health, family involvement in memory care is on the rise as more families than previously believed visit loved ones.[25] Greater accessibility, more flexible work hours, and nicer accommodations have been linked to the upsurge in visits, however, there are still many lonely residents who rarely have visitors.

7.   **Your job title** – While no caregiver would ever ask who you think you are, it is a top complaint among staff who hear far too many complaints from certain family members. The word used is *entitlement*, and it is a hot topic for caregivers. Many family members, who only want the best for their loved one, fail to see the other residents and, because they pay high dollar and visit frequently, feel a sense of entitlement for better, faster treatment than the others there. Fair or not, caregivers try to stay on schedule, on task, and caring for each resident in order.

8.   **We truly appreciate your time** – Family members frequently comment that they want to be liked by the staff or caregivers in hopes of receiving better care for their own loved one. While caregivers work diligently to give equal care, one way to ingratiate yourself to the staff/caregivers is to lend a helping hand. And studies show, a small population of visiting family members do. Caregivers report that many family members become attached to other lonely residents, will bring them gifts, walk with them, or help them when another caregiver is otherwise unavailable. Many will even help in the dining room, handing out drinks or clearing tables so the staff can help the residents. These seemingly small acts of kindness go a long way with caregivers who sometimes feel there is not enough time or love to give to each resident.

9.   **We are family…just not on Facebook** – The people who help care for your loved ones are part of your family. If you do not feel this or believe this is so…this is unfair and

---

[25] Gaugler, J., "Family Involvement in Residential Long-Term Care: A Synthesis and Critical Review," Aging Mental Health. 2005, Mar; 9(2): 105-118. https://www.ncbi.nlm.nih.gov/pmc/articles/PMC2247412/

unreasonable for all concerned. They are. But just as important as it is for you accept this growing family so, took, should you realize there are boundaries. Caregivers (the good ones) give their all at work. Once they leave, however, they need to be able to focus on their own family, friends, and lives. Texting or calling them outside of work, including engaging on their social media accounts, is not okay and not fair to the caregiver.

10.   **A doctor in the house** – Let the trained medical professionals play doctor. Too many loving and well-meaning family members hope to diagnosis and treat symptoms, demanding more or different medications be dispensed. There are exceptions. Many of the stories in this very book describe the overmedication and neglect of some caregivers. In these instances, intervention was necessary. Before you begin calling doctors and nurses during and after hours, demanding new medications, ask other family members and friends to visit your loved one. Get an honest assessment of "Is this normal?" or are you simply trying to find a miracle cure to slow some of the natural processes of dementia. Your medical team *should* be part of the team, not adversaries.

Chapter Twenty-One

Residential Living, Assisted Living, and Memory Care

Already, there have been several references to the amazing Ms. Pat. She was a former neighbor, who later befriended my entire family and became one of the most important women in our mother's life.

For the last sections of this book, "Prepare Your File Folder," and even our own Power of Attorney copy, Ms. Pat was the inspiration.

The day she walked over to my house and announced that she was selling almost everything, house included, and moving, I was astounded. She had lived in her house for as long as anyone could remember and was as healthy as a horse, so where was she going? And why?

Though it seemed spur-of-the-moment to the rest of us, Ms. Pat had been plotting this move for some time. She didn't want to grow "too old" in her own home and leave a mess for others to clean up. She didn't like unfinished business. She knew a time was coming when getting out and about would be more difficult and, she wanted to bring the social aspect of senior living closer to her home. On this one, even the most skeptical of neighbors and friends could only nod and agree. Ms. Pat was extremely social.

She did her research.

She did her due diligence.

She discovered a not-for-profit life-plan communities and services in Ohio[26], based in Columbus, that offers apartment living, assisted living, rehabilitation, and long-term living care. What made this arrangement so perfect was Ms. Pat arranged to move into the apartment living knowing one

---

[26] https://www.ohioliving.org/

day she would have to transition to the assisted and, possibly, long-term care living sections. But because she initially moved into the apartment living area, she also had the option to stay right where she was but utilize the on-site care team.

Leaving home and a life you've always known (aka independence) is the number one reason why senior adults do not willingly move to assisted living or memory care when they most need it. Ms. Pat knew this and wanted to be proactive.

Residential Living

The apartment was perfect for Ms. Pat. She lived in what is called Thurber Tower, which has one hundred and fifty either studio, one-, two-, or three-bedroom apartments, each coming with or without their own balcony. Ms. Pat chose one with a balcony and had our father fasten chicken wire around it so her cats could spend their days outside without her having to worry about them jumping or falling off the balcony.

She signed a contract that stipulated when the time came, she would be able to move into whatever care was needed. Included in her apartment fee were all utilities and Internet, maintenance, twenty-four-hour emergency and security systems, and a fitness center with an on-call personal trainer and a heated pool. A wellness nurse was also on hand as was transportation for community outings, although Ms. Pat continued to drive for another decade after moving into her apartment. She no longer had to worry about trash removal, shoveling snow or lawn maintenance, and Thurber Tower even provided a computer center with on-site tech people who could help her, garden areas, and housekeeping services if she so chose. When she discovered Thurber Tower even had guest suites so out-of-town visitors could come visit, she couldn't wait to share all the educational, cultural, and social events we could all enjoy together.

Besides the art exhibits, craft classes, shuffleboard, and endless card games, there were actual amenities as well. Ms. Pat never really had to go anywhere unless she wanted to. They had a woodshop, banking services, a chapel, art studio, bistro, and library. In fact, there was even a very active book club, which Ms. Pat ultimately convinced Mom she just had to join. It gave Mom and Ms. Pat the chance to get together at least once a month for many, many months.

Assisted Living

Had she transitioned to the assisted-living side, very little would have changed beyond more guidance during day-to-day social events (to keep her active), and the twenty-four-hour personal-care assistance. Things like housekeeping, personal assessment, and care throughout the day would not have been an option but a guarantee.

The idea of assisted living is to provide a personalized care for those who need it.

In truth, had our mother not wanted to join our father in memory care, we would have opted for assisted living for her. While she was also a candidate for memory care, I think she would have been happier in assisted living, with staff available to help her dress and shower and do wellness checks during the day. She would have felt more independent. Mom was just high functioning enough that a security system in play with professional caregivers could have been her life. Because assisted living prepares meals and offers a social setting while being cared for, she might have been able to find a life of her own. For Mom, it was not so much a factor of where she was cognitively but emotionally.

Daddy, however, was the complicated factor.

Recently, I spoke with a woman who moved her mother from assisted living to memory care after caregivers remarked that her mother had begun to wander. The daughter wanted to be proactive in her mother's care and immediately moved her to memory-care living and her

mother's health plummeted.

Rather than have a full assessment of her mother's emotional, cognitive, and physical state, the

daughter believed she was doing the right thing by moving quickly, but it was move not quite

right (at the time) for her mother.

It is important to remember that while dementia is a progressive disease, it is different for every

person. For some, the disease causes rapid decline while others continue to function fairly well

for many years.

For Ms. Pat, this was never an issue. Although I often smile when I think about her comments—

"I'm starting to forget things!"

"You're *ninety*, Ms. Pat! Hell, I've been forgetting things since I was twelve!"

For Ms. Pat, pre-planning for long-term memory care was never needed, but had she needed it,

she would and could have moved to the rehabilitation and long-term nursing care that was also

on-site.

Not everyone has those options.

Be prepared for the costs of long-term care.

According to the 2013 Cost of Care Survey by financial group Genworth, the national median

cost for hourly home care is $19 per hour, whereas costs for adult day health care is $65 per

month. The costs are significantly higher for assisted living. A one-bedroom, single occupancy

averages at $3,450 a month. This includes full-time personal care, including medical. For the

average American, life insurance policies help fund or, at least, help offset such costs.

The cost for long-term memory or nursing homes for a semi-private room runs, average, $207 per day or roughly $6,296.25 per month. A private room in the same type facility averages $230 per day, or approximately $6,995.83 per month.[27]

We do not know how Ms. Pat funded her own long-term care. We do know she had an estate sale, sold her home, and placed the earnings into her new (and forever) home. We know Ms. Pat was unafraid of her own future, and because she was so determined not to be a burden to anyone else, she was able to think through and act upon her "final chapter" plan for her life. So, too, should we all.

---

[27] Executive Summary Genworth 2013 Cost of Care Survey: Home Care Providers, Adult Day Health Care Facilities, Assisted Living Facilities and Nursing Homes. Genworth Financial, Inc. and National Eldercare Referral Systems, LLC (CareScout)**https://www.genworth.com/dam/Americas/US/PDFs/Consumer/corporate/131168_031813_Executive%20Summary.pdf**

Chapter Twenty-Two

#LifeInMemoryCare

After being gone for two full days while he stayed at the VA for observation, Daddy shuffled back into the memory-care facility. He honestly appeared pleased to be there and Londa, the event coordinator and true angel on Earth, saw him, lit up, and exclaimed, "There's my bad boy! I missed him so much. It's been so quiet here!"

Finding A Memory-care Facility

This is an extremely emotional exercise as you are literally placing the care of your loved one into the hands of strangers, walking away, and praying the strangers will be kind. This is your mom, dad, grandparent, aunt or uncle. Maybe this is your husband or wife, which I believe, must be more agonizing than anything else. Therefore, it is all the more important to do your due diligence. Take all the time you need to find the right place for the *entire* family. It is frequently said that there will be no perfect memory-care or assisted-living facility, but you should still have certain expectations and standards.

Ask yourself a few important questions as you begin to tour different facilities.

Memory-care Checklist

❖ **Is it clean?** The facility's standard of cleanliness is a definite indicator of management, how the facility is run, and its own standards of hygiene and cleanliness for its residents.

❖ **Is there a smell?** All too often, people complain about facility's having an "old person smell." A clean facility ought not have this smell, regardless of who the residents are. Something as minor (or major) as smell can and will deter people from visiting.

❖ **Does the staff appear happy?** While visiting a facility, my sister and I noted the staff gave no eye contact, never smiled, and did not speak to the residents. Later, I researched the particular facility and learned the company made a "The 19 Worst Companies to Work For In 2016," list on MSN news as was twelfth on the list for "least happy employees." There is no way the residents were getting the kind of love and joy they needed from caregivers in that kind of environment.[28]

❖ **Do you get a family vibe?** Piggy-backing on the happiness factor, happy employees are essential. When employees are happy, it rolls over to the residents and their families. The single most important reason we chose to put our parents in the facility they are in now is because of the feeling of unity, teamwork, and happiness we felt. One year later, that feeling has only grown.

❖ **Have you looked at comments online or business reports about this care facility?** Again, researching the reputation of a company or a particular facility is important but don't stop there. Get online, look at review sites such as Yelp, Angie's List, Consumer Affairs, Better Business Bureau, Google Reviews, and Glassdoor, to name a few. Do not check one. Check many sites. There will always be unfair reviews, but when you see seventeen reviews discussing poor living conditions, unhappy staff and/or accusations of neglect within the same facility, you are more aware.

❖ **Do *not* take their word.** Placement business, such as A Place for Mom, Aging Matters, or Visiting Angels, are a great place to start, but they are not the be all, end all of memory care. Certainly, listen to their expertise, but do your own research. I described the neglect and abuse my father throughout this story. When I shared that information with a representative from a placement agency, the agent ignored my statements. The agent did not want to hear negative reports that might have a negative impact on her own business. Does this mean the entire company is bad? Not at all. It does, however, show one agent can be negligent in her own duties and ultimately become part of the abuse problem among the elderly.*

❖ **Do the residents appear happy or, at least, comfortable?** Happy is subjective in memory care, but you can gauge how content or comfortable residents are with frequent visits. Are they clean? Do they appear to like their caregivers? A woman who lives alongside our parents in the memory care can be quite surly depending on her level of anxiety. During high anxiety times, we steer clear of her. But she can also be very loving and affectionate, calling people darlin' and sweetie. She walks nonstop, looping the large hallways, and frequently sits on one of the many chairs or padded benches made available through the Isle. Even in her

---

[28] https://www.msn.com/en-us/money/careersandeducation/the-19-worst-companies-to-work-for/ar-BBC0mpH#image=BBC0csU|9

state of dementia and agitation, she is comfortable, well cared for and at ease with her surroundings. In #LifeInMemoryCare world, this is as good as it gets.

❖ **Do the caregivers engage with?** Caregivers who enjoy coming to work, love working with their residents, and are generally happy people will engage in conversation. This doesn't mean there are long sit-down talks about life and politics. But they will look you in the eye, smile, ask how you are doing, and genuinely want to make sure their residents are as happy as they can be.

❖ **Is there an open-door policy?** Ask to visit several times and at different times during the day. Knowing residents' behaviors will change by the hour, do not judge a facility by that behavior but, rather, the overall organization. For example, a visitor came to the memory care to find one of the residents streaking and another yelling at the nude one for streaking. Caregivers were trying to catch the streaker and also calm the streak-offended. All the while, the caregivers were chuckling about the fact that the streaker had mustered up enough energy and chutzpah to streak. They did not worry about the visitor judging them as they were 1) truly amused (in an affectionate manner) by their streaker and 2) pleased to have caught her in time. The visitor was soon smiling, as it was clear there was a lot of love and care in the room. This is #LifeInMemoryCare and they are proud of it. Come one, come all.

❖ **Is it possible for you to talk to other resident families?** Don't be afraid to ask to speak to the families of other residents. You should be able to talk to them privately. Ask their opinion of the facility, how it is run, the treatment of their loved one, and how they came to choose that particular facility. Interestingly, in our case, the facility with a complaint lodged to the state is also one that discouraged management from sharing information between families. My sister and I began finding and talking to people in the parking lot to get answers to certain questions. This should have been our first of *many* red flags. Remember, you are a champion for your loved one.

❖ **How is the location compared to where you live?** Given the urgency in our own personal experience, we initially did not always have a choice where our father was placed. Having lived both near and far away from different facilities, location does matter. No matter what, of course, you have great intentions of visiting and visiting often. But if/when a loved one is an hour away, traffic, holidays, feeling under the weather, just working long hours, and weekends filled with other commitments can make visiting more of a punishment than an act of love. However, you also do not want to choose a facility as a matter of convenience for yourself (or others) at the expense of proper care, cleanliness, professionalism, or happiness.

*Note: With the backing of many within the medical and care profession, I did lodge a formal complaint against the memory-care facility for neglect and abuse, siting multiple examples and witnesses.

**Care Facility Procedure or Availability vs. What Your Loved One Needs:
Our Own Personal Experience**

❖ **Activity director (Events coordinator)** – Prior to our own experiences with various memory-care facilities, we never imagined this position was that important. We could not have been more wrong. The Activity Director, AD, is one of the most important people in the memory-care facility. This person coordinates activities to keep people engaged but also keeps tabs on birthdays, anniversaries, and makes it his/her business to know the back stories of all the residents. The difference in facilities that do and do not have an AD is glaringly apparent. While non-AD facilities are extremely quiet (and, in my opinion, depressing), a facility with an engaged AD is playing BINGO, planning outings, social events, concerts, and crafts.

❖ **Transportation** – We never realized how confining and isolated our father had been until we moved to a facility that had transportation. What a delight it is to come in for a visit only to learn our parents have been out for drives in the country or around town so Daddy could point at and read signs out loud. They listen to the radio and watch the world go by. Daddy loves bus rides. It opened up new kinds of interesting, fun, but safe outings for our parents.

❖ **Food prep and presentation** - After Daddy's fall, food prep and presentation were the last things on our minds. After nearly a year of our parents being fed sandwiches, Cheetos, hot dogs, and macaroni and cheese, however, we now understand the importance of quality food and how it is presented. Our parents now dine with linen napkins, real plates, and flatware but they are also provided nutritional meals as varied and tasty as they are visually appealing. This means so much.

❖ **Design of the building** – The layout of the memory-care facility is a personal preference and something you need to consider for your loved one. For us, our father's ability to walk and walk and walk is crucial. Therefore, he is in a facility with long hallways, an array of furniture he can constantly move and rearrange, colorful pictures, and workstations set up for busy hands. Consider the needs of your loved on in terms of walking and exploring. Additionally, he has access to an enclosed patio, complete with flowers and other attractive foliage, nice patio furniture ready to be rearranged, and a peaceful setting. Outside, there is a walking trail. These may be extremely important amenities to consider.

❖ **Your room** – Navigation has never been an issue for our father. However, our mother has an exceedingly difficult time discerning which room is hers. Facilities should have a method of identifying rooms beyond a nametag since many of those with dementia do not read names. Our parents' room has a shadow box with pictures of family as a reminder for our mother each time she sees familiar faces.

❖ **Security system** – Our father—the man, the myth, the memory-care legend—has certainly tested each and every security system in every facility, hospital, and rehabilitation center we have been in, including the VA. Find out what the security procedures are in regards to locked-in facilities, visitors, in the event of an escape, response to fire alarms, and windows.

❖ **Toilet/tissue policy** – This may seem an obscure item to list, but it is a very real issue. So many residents put tissue and toilet paper into the toilet and then flood the bathroom (because they do know where the tissue goes but don't or can't recall why or when). That's why many caregivers withhold the products. It's understandable, except for higher-functioning adults who can still use the bathroom. Ask about these policies. You know what your loved one is capable of. As long as s/he can still go to the restroom by themselves, you want to encourage this bit of independence, but they must have toilet paper.

❖ **Shower time** – For many people who live with dementia, shower time is frightening. Water or the sensation of water pressure and temperature can actually be painful for many, while others associate showers with the vulnerability of being nude and/or the stripping of clothing. A seemingly innocent act of hygiene can become very traumatic. You need to know what the procedures are for bathing. Our own father became aggressive as a defense against what we're sure he saw as a violation and, thus, the need to protect himself. It was not until we moved to a new facility and new tactics were used that our father became comfortable with bathing again. Shower time is one event that cannot be rushed or forced.

❖ **Alone time and what that means to caregivers** – Alone time is something our father lives for. He likes to be alone, exploring and wandering. For many people with dementia, the sounds of everyday activities can be overwhelming. The dining hall, the activity room, even normal conversation can be too much, and many Alzheimer's and dementia patients just want/need time alone. Many caregivers are secretly relieved by this as they can then turn their attention to the nineteen other things needing their attention. But how much time are residents given? How long will they remain alone before someone checks on them and does anyone note if the alone time appears to increase?

❖ **Distribution of medication** – Every person is different. For some, the onset of sundowning (a term used for *late-day confusion* for those with Alzheimer's and other forms of dementia) comes at different times. For our parents, we learned their evening medications (to help with sleep) comes at 7 pm. By 2 am, they were awake and terrorizing the halls. Adjusting the times your loved one takes certain medications can help alleviate some behavioral issues. This said, many facilities and the nursing staff work very hard to stay on a set schedule and do not like to vary.

While considering how the facility best suits your loved one, the reality is it should be a comfortable fit with you as well. In the **Memory-care Checklist**, you were asked to consider drive time and travel convenience as well as rating the family vibe feeling. These are important for you and your loved ones, but there are some extra considerations for you to keep in mind as well. Not only do you want your loved one to be comfortable, but you need to find a place that feels authentic for you too.

How the Facility Rates for You, The Loved One, and Caregiver:
More Things to Consider

❖ **Does this feel like family?** You were asked this in regards to how caregivers behave with your loved one, but what about you? Recently, a woman posted that she hated visiting her mother in a care facility because "I know they [caregivers] all hate me. I'm always asking for things, and they can't stand me." This is a big problem. You don't have to be great buddies but there does need to be a camaraderie between you and the caregivers. Any animosity is a red flag. If it cannot be resolved, this is not the facility for you or your loved one.

❖ **Do you feel trust or uneasiness?** Trust is a big issue in the care industry. You can and should take certain precautions. To head off any problems, we took our parents fine jewelry since the likelihood of Mom losing her valuables then blaming caregivers was excellent. But if you have feelings of neglect, abuse, theft, etc., it must be addressed immediately.

❖ **Do they call you? Will they call you?** Whether you are still checking out different facilities or have moved into one, it is good to know what their policies are about making calls. Let them know you love text messages and pictures updating you on how well your loved one is doing, but you also don't mind getting a call if your loved one is suddenly scared or confused. Let this new team know you are available even when you are not present.

❖ **When will they call you? Why will they call you?** But, and there is a *but.*, make sure the reason for contacting you is appropriate. Early on, some caregivers discovered if they called us saying, "Your father is out of control," we would come running. Before we knew it, we were handling our father's most difficult behaviors all hours of the day and night. It must be clear that you cannot take phone calls at all hours because a caregiver does not want to handle the more difficult behaviors. That is not your job, but theirs.

❖ **How about sleepovers**? If you want or need to spend the night with your loved on, is this a possibility for you?

❖ **What is there for *you* at the facility?** Again, my sister and I joke we're memory-care experts after being in the big and small, corporate and private, facilities and homes. We've been there at all hours, overnight, during holidays, and on the weekends. You never know what dementia will deliver and so it is nice to have a place where you can work from the facility, get coffee, grab something to eat, watch TV, curl up on a couch, help with other residents, or walk with your loved one. You are more likely to visit and stay if the facility is welcoming to you and your needs as well. This doesn't mean you should camp out there but in the wee hours of the morning, it is nice to have some accommodations.

❖ **What about the pets?** Many facilities are now using pet therapy for their residents with wonderful results. But what about your loved one's pet? Is it permissible for Fluffy to come for a visit (assuming Fluffy is well behaved)? You never know unless you ask. Find out the policy for short visits with four-legged family members.

❖ **Is there access to caregivers, executive directors, and/or owners?** As previously detailed, we lost all communication with the director of a former facility when plumbing issues caused flooding in our parents' room and again when there were safety issues with the staff's treatment of our parents. These were not small but very dangerous and costly problems and yet we got no response. You need assurances. If there were a medical and family emergency or a true concern about safety, you must be able to speak to someone to rectify the problem. This is not an unreasonable expectation as your loved one cannot fend for him/herself.

❖ **What about medical information**? This is not an uncommon concern/complaint among family members who are suddenly concerned about new or odd behavior and cannot gain insight into what medications are being dispensed and how often. Your new facility should make medical information available to you upon request.

❖ **Is the facility part of the community**? An active facility is an engaged facility. As a business model, it is great marketing, but this also bodes well for you and your loved one. As a community gets to know a facility, in this case, people pay more attention to the business, its employees, and its residents. Case in point: Because our facility is known for its communal efforts, it was the facility contacted by the Alzheimer's Association and how we became active in the walk.

Chapter Twenty-Three

The Everything File: Learning the Hard Way

This chapter was probably the most difficult to write as all of the following information was learned the hard way. This was also the first chapter written.

Prepare Your File Folder of Information (aka The Everything File):

(These forms should all be copies with the originals kept in a safe or secure place)

- ❖ Birth certificate
- ❖ Driver's license
- ❖ Social security card
- ❖ Passport
- ❖ Marriage license (if applicable)
- ❖ Tax returns for the past two years
- ❖ Bank – list any and all banks you have accounts with, list the type of accounts (saving and/or checking), including account number, routing number, addresses, phone numbers, and the name of your point of contact within each bank.
- ❖ Medical – includes a list of doctors along with addresses and phone number, medical information/history, all medications, any allergies, and hospital stays (if any)
  - ➢ Your Power of Attorney, another family member, and your physician should all meet, be familiar with each other, and have an understanding of your long-term wants and needs, be it a retirement center, memory-care facility, hospice, and/or funeral arrangements.
- ❖ Medical Power of Attorney – Be sure you have signed the proper HIPAA forms allowing your POA and one other family member to gather medical information in the event you can no longer give consent.
  - ➢ The Medical Power of Attorney should state that, in the event you are incapacitated and/or unable to care for yourself, you POA—as described—is legally allowed to make medical decisions for you. This should be signed by a lawyer and the doctor. This will be incredibly helpful to us when we have to move our father into hospice.

❖ <u>Legal</u> – includes the name of the law firm, the attorney used, address, and phone number of the firm. If possible, introduce your named POA to the lawyer.

❖ <u>Power of Attorney paperwork</u> – **critical** Be sure to have Power of Attorney paperwork that is legal and binding. This POA is what will allow your designated family member or friend to carry out your legal and medical plans, to access your accounts and take care of you. Please be sure that it is a POA that allows your designated person access to your bank, financial and medical records.

➢ Have at least two copies in the file. No doubt, your POA will have to make many more over time.

➢ Have this document certified at your local county courthouse, typically within the Department of Records.

❖ <u>Letter of Permission</u> – a letter that offers an explanation of who your POA is and how you hope to have them help you when or in the event that you are unable to care for yourself or your own personal affairs. Having such a letter would have been incredibly helpful to us as we unearthed new accounts and passwords for our parents. While not legally binding, this letter, in conjunction with the POA, can solve and resolve many issues.

❖ <u>If you create a Do-It-Yourself will</u> (not recommended for court reasons as far too many banks and institutions will challenge its validity, and in the long run, this can be costlier and far more time consuming), either have a lawyer look at it or, at the very least, take it to the county courthouse where you live to have it certified.

❖ <u>Make introductions</u> – One of the best things Ms. Pat did was bringing her nephew into each bank she did business with and introducing him to every manager as her POA.

❖ <u>Make your intentions known</u> – If you want to give your POA full access to your accounts or simply want him/her to manage a specific account, list your wants and needs. Is the introduction binding for the bank manager? No. But when bank officials know a person and their intentions, it speeds up the process of inquiry and investigation when your POA comes in with the necessary paperwork. Some institutions with note the verified documentation on your account long before anything happens so much of this can be skipped when the time comes. Check with your bank.

❖ <u>Online Information</u> – list all passwords and security key passwords. *In the event that the Power of Attorney paperwork is not immediately accepted by the legal department of the bank, your POA still has access to your account and can stop any illegal or suspicious activities by logging on-line as you. (While we awaited approval, more than $50,000 was taken from our parents' accounts).

<u>In the event of death</u>: *Note: In no way do I condone this but am only passing along information* As POA for my parents, I was given "behind the scenes" advice from a banker. In the event of my parents' death, a bank must temporarily close down the account while awaiting legal final action from courts. In the meantime, however, bills needing payment are left either to go into default or be paid by the POA or others out of pocket. The advice was to move the money to another active account capable of handling the bills and then notify the bank of the person's death.

Other family members have added to this advice: Social Security moves quickly in the event of a death and banks are instantly notified. Make sure your POA understands that getting to the bank quickly should be a top priority. It is harsh but it is very real.

Note: Passwords and security codes should not be given out prior to illness, injury, or death. These are listed in your "everything file" that your POA has access to when needed.

❖ List the mortgage company, bank (if any), and home insurer of your home and any other properties you own.

❖ Your Power of Attorney should meet with your mortgage lender. An easy drop-by meet and explanation of the introduction can be as quick as five minutes but it is helpful for your mortgage lender and POA to have a face-to-face.

❖ What is the long-term plan for your home?
  ➢ Will it be kept in the family, rented out, or sold?
  ➢ Do you want/need someone to stay in your house?
  ➢ Are there any concerns about break-ins should the house remain vacant for days? Weeks? Months?
  ➢ Will a real estate agent be needed right away for the sale of your home?
  ➢ If you are receiving a newspaper, have you supplied contact to have this shut down?

- ➤ Will you need to contract someone to keep the lawn mowed, lights turned off/on?
- ➤ If you have lawn service, do you wish for this to continue or be stopped? If stopped, include contact information.

- ❖ List all electric, gas (if applicable), water, and trash utility companies you have each month.

- ❖ Make a copy of each (most recent) bill from each utility company and note how each bill is paid. Do you pay by way of check or credit card? Be precise and clear in your notes.

- ❖ Your electronics: List all the phone, Internet, television, and/or cable companies used in your home.

- ❖ Make a copy of each (most recent) bill from each company and note how each bill is paid. Do you pay by way of check or credit card? Be precise and clear in your notes.

- ❖ If you have online accounts, spell out how to get onto your online account, including passwords, usernames, and answers to any security questions. For example, while getting into our father's account with one company, we were asked—for added security—to name the name of his best man at his wedding. We had *no idea*!

Note: Passwords and security codes should not be given out prior to illness, injury, or death. These are listed in your "everything file" that your POA has access to when needed.

- ❖ List all vehicles registered in your name, including make and model, year, color, and condition of vehicle. Sadly, this is one of the first items family and extended family will help themselves to when a loved one is hospitalized, placed in a long-term care facility, or upon death.

- ❖ Have a copy of the title to each vehicle. We were unable to locate the title for our father's car and, because he had moved from Virginia to Texas, it turned into a very long and complicated legal matter. Make sure your title is accessible to your POA.

- ❖ Payment booklet. If you do not own and are still paying on the car, have this information accessible.

- ❖ While this is most likely included in your list of monthly bills, supply of copy of your insurance information and agent with the care title.

- ❖ Any information and bills/receipts you may have regarding the car's history, including tune-up and accidents, should be included for the purpose of resale if/when needed.

❖ Who gets the car? Perhaps you have decided to gift (or sell with the proceeds going toward your estate) to a friend or family member. Make this clear both in writing but also to your POA.

❖ List both major credit cards (American Express, Discover, VISA, and MasterCard) and individual store cards (such as Target, Macy's, Sears, J C Penny's), as well as gas station cards. Debit cards should be listed with your bank information.

❖ If you have online accounts with any/all of the cards, spell out how to sign into your account, including passwords, usernames, and answers to any security questions.

❖ Detail how the cards are paid each month. Check? Online savings? Again, if this is online, be sure your POA has access to passwords and security questions.

Note: Passwords and security codes should not be given out prior to illness, injury, or death. These are listed in your "everything file" that your POA has access to when needed.

❖ List all online accounts you use, whether for shopping, entering contests, job employment opportunities, getting the news, or for social media. Creating a list of church groups can also be helpful to your POA later when he or she is looking for help with different matters involving you, your house, even possible lawn work while you are hospitalized. Remember, even the most seemingly minor account can be a financial and legal headache for your family. Take your time as you compile what could be a lengthy list.

   ➤ Do you use email, such as Gmail, Yahoo, AOL, etc.?

   ➤ Facebook? LinkedIn? Skype? Tumblr?

   ➤ List all the newspaper and/or magazine accounts you may have.

   ➤ List all resale or shopping sites, such as Amazon.com, Apple, iTunes, and any stores you might get coupons or alerts from.

   ➤ Contests, score ratings for credit, and/or charities and organizations you have given to in the past or present.

   ➤ Include your username and passwords, and account numbers for *each* account.

Note: Passwords and security codes should not be given out prior to illness, injury or death. These are listed in your "everything file" that your POA has access to when needed.

❖ List names of all organizations, charities, churches, and/or politicians you have donated monies or provided personal information.

ALERT! ALERT! This is a very important list to compile as your POA may be butting heads with a group that, as good as your intentions or experiences with them were, makes an automatic withdrawal from a bank account you set up two years ago. This is not uncommon. With business and legal out of the way, there are a few more issues you want to address for this file and for your POA. Earlier, we asked, "what does your team roster look like? In the event that you are hospitalized, can no longer take care of yourself, or are deceased, you'll want certain people contacted. Because, let's be honest, you have friends who happen to live in the neighborhood and then you have neighbors. There is a difference. While your POA will contact those you have identified as neighbor friends, there will be many more neighbors wondering about the inactivity or new activity at your house. Depending on your neighborhood and/or relations, you may have special instructions for your POA.

Your POA may not be familiar with all of your friends so help out with a detailed list of names, addresses, and phone numbers. Even more helpful, note how you know this person and if there is any special information you want passed along to a particular friend. This list includes:

➤ Neighborhood friends
➤ Gym friends
➤ Church friends
➤ Senior center friends
➤ Social media buddies
➤ Distant relatives and old friends whom you do not see regularly but share correspondence with.

List your pets, including ages, the name of your veterinarian, medications taken, brand of food, and the daily schedule—from eating times to possible walks, favorite play toys, and car rides.

This list will ensure your POA knows to gather up favorite toys, bedding, leashes, bowls, and medical files for the new owner or short-term babysitter if you are hospitalized.

You should already know who you want to take your pet(s). This should not be a job for your POA. Have the name and contact information of who has agreed to take your animals. Have a realistic talk with this person so they understand what challenges they may be undertaking and them introduce your POA with the person(s) who has agreed to take on Fluffy and/or Fido.

Finally—how do you want your personal items handled?

Ms. Pat had an estate sale and had the great joy of watching her friends, family, neighbors, and fellow church members, whom she loved, choose and then cherish the one-of-a-kind Ms. Pat items. The beauty of it all was that this was her call. This was all her choice.

For us, however…we missed out on that particular joy. For us, this is taking care of business. While Mom and Daddy are still with us, many things remain in the house, but Michelle and I have created a list of things we hope to give to our parents' surviving family when the time comes. Until then, as detailed previously, Michelle and I had family pick and choose between various items in the house. We knew our Uncle Stephen would appreciate old tools our father had that once belonged to their father (our grandfather). An antique school desk, for example, went to a cousin who is also an educator. We then had a garage sale for items, such as kitchenware and trinkets from around the world, no one else wanted.

Make a list of the things you most care about and designate who gets what. Believe it or not, this is more for your POA than you. It is a particularly difficult task—filled with guilt and second-guessing, sadness and concern—but a crucial one. When the list is made, create copies for everyone.

We heard many stories in which, following the death of a parent, one sibling entered the home unbeknownst to the others and helped himself to family treasures before anyone else could be there. If you compile and list and make it known to family and friends, it makes those behaviors less likely.

What Are Family Treasures?

- ❖ Furniture and artwork
- ❖ Jewelry
- ❖ Crystal, china, silver(ware)
- ❖ Pictures, photo albums, and family records
- ❖ Personal letters, cards, and journals
- ❖ Antiques/family heirlooms, including items such as a handmade blanket by Grandmother, doilies passed down from generation to generation, etc.
- ❖ Collectibles and souvenirs
- ❖ Books
- ❖ Electronics and appliances that may have some significance to a particular person but, if left unidentified, could easily be given away in a garage sale or to a thrift store
- ❖ Clothing, including particular coats, ties, dresses, etc. you want to go to a very specific person.
- ❖ Tools and/or machinery, including lawn mower. As astonishing as this may sound, there are family members who will come into a home to take a washer and dryer while their loved one is in memory care or just passed. Identify these larger and expensive items.
  - ➢ Do all major appliances stay with the home?
  - ➢ Are they sold and the proceeds going to the estate?
  - ➢ Have you promised them to a specific person, family member, or organization?
- ❖ Bikes, cars, and any other motorized vehicles.
- ❖ Houseplants

Chapter Twenty-Four

The Last Chapter

My Uncle Stephen, Michelle, and I took Daddy to the VA. The idea was to have the neurologists monitor Daddy's level of brain damage. As always, they think they can talk to him.

VA rep: Do you know where you are and why you're here, sir?

Daddy: [reaches over and flips off a light switch and we all sit in the dark for a moment, and then he flips it back on.]

Light off.

Yup. This pretty much wraps up our last year.

Light on.

But things have dramatically improved.

Light off.

It's just so hard.

Light on.

He nodded, satisfied, and let the light remain on.

That seems about right.

Many years ago, I wrote a murder mystery that had more readers than not confessing, "I had no idea who it was until the very end." As an author, I cannot brag on this literary bit of mystery achievement since I didn't know either! That admission always gets a chuckle, but it's no less true. I really didn't. I just let the characters take me to the very end.

And when I was pregnant with my first child, I opted out of the whole Lamaze-prepare-yourself-for-what's-coming thing and decided I would wing it. I mean…women have been winging childbirth for centuries, right? How hard could it be?

It was hard.

But this business with my parents, having to face their eventual deaths while they are blissfully unaware, has been the hardest thing yet, and I cannot wing this or let the moment carry me along. I have to be like Ms. Pat.

I have too many questions. For example, I know my maternal grandparents purchased a three-grave plot in St. Joseph, Missouri, where both maternal grandparents are laid to rest, but what am

I supposed to do with that third plot? Is there paperwork somewhere? I can't even remember the name of the cemetery. I can only remember Mom scoffing at the notion that she would be buried with her parents and not her husband.

I have always known Daddy wanted to be buried in Arlington Cemetery, with full honors. But where does that leave Mom?

I know Mom wants to be cremated, but what about Daddy?

When a friend of my father's mentioned Arlington Cemetery was experiencing a few *problems*, I did a little research and found some disturbing news. The historic cemetery was running out of room.

I thought it prudent to begin my father's paperwork to apply for a space, not really understanding what was involved, and immediately hit my first wall—I need specific military paperwork I have never been able to find. The missing infamous DD 214 form has been the bane of my existence. Thus far, using my POA, I've managed to wiggle around it.

Back to the VA I go, to yet another department, to start another battle.

Had Daddy placed his military paperwork in one file, perhaps much time and energy and massive tears of hair-ripping frustration could have been spared.

And so, as unpleasant as this subject is, it must be addressed.

The Final Plans

No one simply dies anymore. You can't. It's impossible.

There are two certain facts about death. First, upon your death, many factors (beyond the grief of your loved ones) will come into play with medical, financial, and legal institutions, and second, your POA/executor will be taking care of it all. Therefore, it is time.

First, make funeral arrangements –As unpleasant as this all is, do you really want this to fall on the shoulders of your POA, executor, and/or family members. What may seem like the simplest questions in the world to you can be deflating to others once you're gone. Provide the answers now.

Second, include your POA and/or executor in everything! This can be made easier by simply reviewing this chapter together with your POA.

Ten Funeral Questions You Need to Ask:

1. Do you want to be buried or cremated?

2. Where do you hope to be buried or have your ashes kept? If you want to be buried, do you have a particular headstone in mind? And have you thought about what you would like displayed on it?

3. Do you have a person(s) in mind for who will handle your funeral? Does this person know? Does this person know where your personal, financial, and medical information are kept?

4. How much money do you want spent on your funeral? Before you answer, look at the next section, **The Cost of Dying**.

5. Is there a particular church where you would like to have a service? Do you want a memorial service? A common misconception about funeral directors is that they are clergy and can perform services. They are not and do not. Read **Top Ten Things to Consider About Funeral Homes**.

6. Have you identified a funeral director and/or funeral home yet? This is important and requires interviewing several people. The funeral director who helps your loved one and makes final arrangements for you is incredibly important, not just for you but for your POA and family. If the director has already met—however briefly—with you, he/she will already have a fair idea of what you wanted and what your costs are. They will be less likely to strong-arm or upsell unnecessary packages.

7. Do you know which pictures you want displayed at your funeral? Find ones that showcase your life. This step has been identified as one of the more stressful tasks in planning process. With so many photographs, so little time, and all the memories attached to each one, the challenge can be overwhelming. More importantly, your loved ones will be happier knowing that the pictures displayed are special to you.

8. Ever thought about writing your own eulogy? If not, perhaps you can make a list of things you are most proud of in your life. This can include children and grandchildren, previous jobs, travels, churches, and organizations you belonged to, hobbies, even a list of "Ten things we bet you didn't know about Cousin Lulu!"

   More people than you imagine involuntarily laugh at funerals. Not because the situation is funny but because when we become so distressed and anxiety filled, laughter is the response mechanism. It is quite common and, for that reason, experts suggest incorporating more laughter into funeral services. It is a celebration of one's life, right? Offer stories of hope, laughter, and light.

9. Who do you want at your funeral? This is a very difficult question, but it deserves an answer. If you don't, someone else has to. Do you care who the pallbearers are? Who might sing and which song? Who will speak?

10. What will you wear? However morbid this may seem, if there is something, let people know. Make it clear that you have a uniform, a favorite suit or dress that you want to be buried in. This answer, however trivial it may seem to you right now, can be a devastating decision for a grieving family member.

The Cost of Dying

The cost of a funeral is more expensive than ever but so, too, is the act of dying. According to the National Bureau of Economic Research, out-of-pocket expenditures leading up to and upon death average $11,618 per person. Of course, those numbers fluctuate wildly, especially when you start looking at the average funeral cost running $5,166 and the average medical costs associated with dying costing $9,875. Additionally, the National Funeral Directors Association estimates that the median out-of-pocket funeral costs are $6,078 per person.

Even the states where the death certificate is issued vary. For example, the state of Mississippi has no estate tax or inheritance tax, which is why it's the least expensive of all the states in the United States in terms of cost associated with dying.

As we all know, every state has different laws, which translates across the board, including different costs of living and dying. Based on the cost of living index in each state, the Tax Foundation calculated the cost of dying for that state. In 2017, the Tax Foundation included inheritance tax and estate tax data where it applied. The three most expensive states are Alaska, (average funeral cost almost $8,000, but medical expenses associated with dying are approximately $15,278), California (the second most expensive state to die in, with funeral costs at $8,284 and medical expenses associated with dying close to $16,000), and Hawaii (funeral costs run over $11,000 and medical costs associated with end-of-life care close to $22,000).[29] Be aware of the costs of your state, including inheritance and estate taxes.

---

[29] DePietro, A. The Cost of Dying in Each State, GOBankingRates. http://www.msn.com/en-us/money/personalfinance/the-cost-of-dying-in-each-state/ss-AApi0GT?li=BBnb7Kz#image=1

Thirteen Things to Consider When Looking at Funeral Homes

The funeral industry is both a noble and necessary profession but, like anything else, there are a few bad apples spoiling the bunch if you aren't careful.

1. **Check credentials** – Check out the funeral home before you even check it out. That is, check with your state's board of funeral directors or contact the National Funeral Directors Association (NFDA) to gather more information. The NFDA is an advocate for you, "dedicated to supporting members in their mission to provide families with meaningful end-of-life services at the highest levels of excellence and integrity." Check out www.nfda.org, or the Funeral Consumers Alliance, another organization committed to ensuring that "consumers are fully prepared and protected when planning a funeral," at www.funerals.org.

2. **Pay-on-death account** – Many consumer advocates warn against paying funeral homes in advance as you could lose everything if a funeral home goes out of business. Instead, banks offer a 'Payable-on-Death' accounts that keep your money out of probate. Talk to your bank to learn more. Briefly, this account has you name who you want to inherit the money in the account or certificate of deposit. The bank and the beneficiary (who may or may not be the POA) can then bypass probate court and pay all bills on time.

3. **Veterans** – For those who have served and/or their spouses, burial is free at the Veterans Affairs National Cemetery. This includes the grave/vault, opening and closing, the marker, and setting fee. Contact the VA for more information as many of the state veterans' cemeteries also offer free burial for veterans and, often, spouses (www.cem.va.gov).

4. **The cost of caskets** – You do not have to pay full price for a casket through a funeral home. Caskets can also be purchased online from Walmart, Costco, or from the manufacturer. You should also know that a funeral provider cannot refuse or charge a fee to handle a casket you bought somewhere else. That is federal law.

5. **Skip the package deals** – According to financial and banking sources, these so-called package deals are no deals at all. During a time of grief and/or crisis, most people readily agree to whatever appears easiest and most convenient. In such packages, consumers are

frequently sold ideas that simply are not true or hidden within the small print. You need to see everything itemized to know what you are paying for.

6. **Embalming** – The United States and Canada are the only countries in the world to regularly embalm the deceased. Consumers are told that it is for public health, despite evidence to the contrary. For funeral homes that have a refrigeration room—which most should have—there is no reason to embalm, elevating the extra expense that will run between $500 and $1200.

7. **Funeral Consumer Alliance (FCA)** – Funeral directors might refuse to have a public viewing without embalming, but this is not a legal requirement (except in Minnesota). Check with the FCA on your rights.

8. **Sealed—aka *expensive*—caskets are best for preserving the body** – This is another myth.[30]

9. **Not every funeral service is the same** – Prices for funeral homes can vary greatly, with cremation costs starting at $500 and going as high as $3,000 between two seemingly similar funeral homes. Do not be afraid to bargain hunt. The terms *bargain* and *funeral* make most people feel uneasy, and that is what funeral homes bank on.

10. **Over-the-phone pricing** – Federal law **_requires_** prices be provided over the phone upon request. A funeral home may try to tell you that you must come in, but this is untrue, punishable, and must be reported.

11. **Where to have the service** – This is your choice. It does not have to be at a funeral home. It can be in a church, your home, a community center, or even a local park. Many families opt for more personal settings, thus saving thousands of dollars for the more direct burial or direct cremation involving no embalming, viewing, or visitation. For memorials, it is suggested that family print memorial cards, decorate a room with pictures and notes, or even use a PowerPoint presentation of pictures and favorite expressions used by the deceased.

12. **Do this for your loved one** – Funeral directors offer a wonderful service but many take more of a salesman approach to peddle their varied services. In a time of great

---

[30] Goodstein, E. "10 Things Funeral Directors Don't Want You To Know," Bankrate.com. http://www.bankrate.com/finance/jobs-careers/things-funeral-directors-dont-want-you-to-know.aspx#ixzz4q947e3DD

vulnerability, families often hear, "This is the last wonderful thing you can do for your loved one," and it's typically followed by a mighty price tag. Whether you are pre-planning your own funeral or doing this for a loved one, think about what you want to spend. More money spent doesn't equal better. It just means more money spent.

13. **Do not visit funeral homes alone** – Again, whether you are making pre-planning or doing this for a loved one who is now deceased, do not go alone. This is an emotional and difficult task. Visiting funeral homes and talking to directors requires many ears. Do not commit to anything upon the initial visit and take detailed notes for later discussion. This is the one place where the "do this for your loved one," statement is most appropriate.

"I never saw a dollar bill cry at anyone's funeral."

– J. Lincoln Fenn

What Are You Waiting For?

Preferably, this is the job of the person in question, but like many things, once this is no longer an option, it falls to the POA. Remember, one plans on face-planting onto the kitchen floor about as often as they plan on dementia, and that would be *never*.

This chapter opened with the story of my father and his one known request to be buried in Arlington Cemetery. As of this writing, having successfully petitioned to acquire his Honorable Discharge paperwork and his DD 214 form from the National Personnel Records Center in St. Louis, I now await paperwork submitted to the Arlington Cemetery.

While one could argue that the paperwork should have been placed into a file for easy access, what would be the point? That proverbial ship has sailed so…now it is in the hands of the POA—me.

At present, my father's health is relatively good. He is ambulatory (too much, some would argue), has a great appetite (too much, some would argue), and probably more content now than he has been in the past year. Still, my job as POA is to have everything lined up, so I am being proactive.

It is human nature to put off those things that are most unpleasant and planning a funeral tops the list. While I have often found myself feeling more saddened than burdened in this task, I know two things:

1. It has to be done. At some point, this is a non-negotiable task to be performed.

2. It will be worse if I wait.

As *Operation Caregivers: #LifewithDementia* entered the final stages of editing, one of my favorite Silver Sneaker students approached me in the gym. She was also one of my readers and took the checklist to heart.

"I wanted you to know I've done everything on the list," Dorothy Baysore said, adding that she has also decided to arrange her own funeral.

Why?

Simple. She did not want to leave that task to her children and grandchildren. She said the hardest part was not arranging her own funeral but, rather, the memories of arranging the funerals of both of her parents and her husband.

When I asked if she was glad she'd done it, she did not hesitate.

"Yes!"

For Dorothy, now knowing her children will not have to make all the difficult decisions—what casket, what kind of service, and where—was a relief.

As discussed again and again in this very book, however, there are always new challenges one cannot plan for.

Dorothy experienced that very thing while sitting in the funeral home, making arrangements for her burial plot. Years earlier, her husband was cremated. and together they agreed that he (his urn) would be buried with her. It's a beautiful idea. But when she mentioned this at the funeral home, while laying out the details of her plan, she learned that she would have to buy two plots because, legally, there could not be two people in a single plot.

"I argued and argued," she said, dejectedly. In the end, however, she was forced to buy a second plot.

Legally speaking, this is only partially true. Depending upon the cemetery's policy, there are different ways in which an urn/the cremated loved one can be buried with a casketed loved one. Many cemeteries will allow for cremains to be buried on top of the casket. Still, there are also cemeteries that do allow the urn to be placed inside the casket and do not require a second gravesite. Just as we've discussed in other scenarios, this legal issue varies from state to state, and from cemetery to cemetery. Know the policies of your state and cemetery of choice.

In the case of Robb's cousin, Duane Sessions, he has it all figured out. Still very young, healthy, and strong, I was surprised to hear him announce his teenage daughter would be planning his funeral. An avid sportsman and hunter, Duane declared that Amy, fourteen years old, would do something "cool."

"So, there's two options. Option #1, have me taxidermized so that she can still drive around with me and have someone to talk to all the time. She concerned that this might be illegal, however, so Option #2 is to cremate me, mix me with gunpowder and load me into shotgun shells so she can quite literally take me hunting me. We brainstorm other ideas whenever it's just the two of us but those are our favorites right now."

Legalities aside, they talk about it. While hilarious and morbid, this list of ideas also serves as a great reminder about funerals and the planning of. Every person is different. For some, the traditional funeral is just that—traditional and right. For others, a simple memorial, with a small gathering of friends, perhaps a photo gallery showing adventures and milestones, along with a few good stories, is all they want. Still, others want what is popularly known as a "celebration of life," complete with a party. As this section is so titled, this is *your* last chapter. Make your wishes known.

Delegating Tasks

Earlier, we discussed having a team, and believe me when I say, people want to help. This is a perfect time to pull out the roster and assign positions. Whether it is for your life or you are the POA, it's time to delegate. Put out some feelers to see who would like to have a role in planning and putting into action things needed for a funeral. Once you have a list, assign the tasks, then send everyone a copy so each person knows what the others are doing. This network will prevent people from tripping over each other but also allows them to team up on some tasks.

Checklist of Common Tasks

1. Who will arrange refreshments and drinks?

2. Who will be in charge of flowers, cards, and all charitable donations made in honor of you/your loved one?

3. Who will arrange the phone tree letting people know what, when, and where concerning any functions—the funeral, celebration of life, family get-together?

4. Who will be in charge of pictures, quotes, and cards for the memory/honorary display?

5. Who will be responsible for organizing and/or delivering the eulogy? If there are multiple speakers, one person should be in charge of who is speaking and when.

6. Who will be in charge of printing/publishing the obituary? This includes deciding ahead of time which publications, social media sites, newsletters, and/or organizations to be notified of the passing and funeral arrangements.

7. Who will be in charge of bringing the clothes for you/your loved one for the funeral service (if this is needed)?

8. Who will take care of pets? The house? Other properties during the funeral and in the days following for the surviving family?

9. Who is taking care of the family? This is a very important detail. Find several people who are willing to take on the role of caring for family. This person/group will do last minute errands, retrieve forgotten items, hold phones and purses, and be ready for the moral support that will be needed.

Write Your Own Obituary

Well before our lives turned upside down, before I ever suspected my mother had Alzheimer's or my father would succumb to dementia, I declared everything I do is for my obituary. As I climbed into a bobsled with a brand new driver who looked so terrified I had no hope for a smooth ride, I looked over my shoulder to a crewmember and said, "Just tell people how confident I looked before we went down the mountain." When I test drove the Volvo Gravity car right before the brakes went out on a mountain that T-boned into an extremely busy intersection, I told Michelle, "I have no regrets!" And just before I dove into the ocean to join my sister and daughters shark diving in open waters with bull sharks, my last words were, "God, I hope these aren't my last words!"

There are two very important aspects to successful obituary-ing.

1.   Get the facts and give the facts

2.   Make your statement

Make Your Statement Yours

Many people struggle with the concept of a funeral being a celebration of a life rather than a death. It is easy enough to say these words until you are saying goodbye to your loved one. The finality of it all can overwhelm everything else.

In writing your own obituary, not only do you have the last say in your life but also in how your loved ones remember that final goodbye. If you are the POA, writing a strong obituary will both honor your charge but also help those grieving the loss.

What do you want to say?

How do you want you or your loved one remembered?

In early 2017, a Wisconsin doctor named Kay Ann Heggestad wrote her own obituary, revealing that she had lost a two-year battle to cancer and imploring her mourners not to say she had *fought a courageous battle*, because she had not! In her words, "she complained all the way."

Prior to his own death in 2014, Walter Bruhl Jr. penned his own obit with fill-in-the-blank sections and bits of humor throughout. "There will be no viewing since his wife refuses to honor his request to have him standing in the corner of the room with a glass of Jack Daniels in his hand so he would appear natural to visitors." Bruhl also noted that he was preceded in death by his tonsils and adenoids, a spinal disc, a large piece of his thyroid gland, and his prostate. He added that, rather than sending flowers to his funeral, he wished his friends and family would perform random acts of kindness "for some poor soul" in his honor.[31]

Perhaps there is no funnier—and telling—obituary than that of Jean Oddi, a ninety-one-year-old woman from Ohio, who wrote, "I hate to admit it, but evidently I died. I'm leaving behind a hell of a lot of stuff."

The raucous, unapologetic obit went viral on social media, triggering hundreds of strangers to reach out to Oddi's family with messages:

"I didn't know you, Jean, but I sure wish I had!"

"I didn't know this gal, but I love her! I can only hope I can live life like she did and go out that way."

For Oddi's family, the obituary and the response it received were healing.[32]

For those who do not have or want humor during such serious times, paying tribute to a life lived well can be done through stories of service, be it with the military, in the community, or within your own family. This is your life's story to tell.

---

[31] Emling, S., "5 Hilarious Obits that Absolutely Killed It," AARP. April 17, 2017.

[32] https://www.ksat.com/inside-edition/hilarious-sassy-obit-goes-viral-i-hate-to-admit-it-but-evidently-i-died_

Get the Facts—Top Ten Things You Want in the Obituary

1. Given name this should also include nicknames, if there are any, but make sure that the proper formal birth name is presented

2. Birth date and place of birth

3. Offer both mother's maiden name, father's name, and their places of birth

4. Occupation and employer(s)

5. Armed service and rank, if applicable

6. Names of those who proceeded your loved one in death

7. Names of survivors and their relationship to your loved one

8. Schools attended and any academic accomplishment/awards worth mentioning

9. Lifetime achievements and/or hobbies

10. List information about the memorial service and funeral (times, locations). Be sure to include specific details about charities if there are memorial donations.

Keep in mind, as hard as this may be, if you are reading this and making life and death decisions for your surviving family members, this is one of the grandest and most selfless things you can do. Just as we marvel at Ms. Pat's foresight and thoughtfulness, so, too, will your loved ones.

Postscript

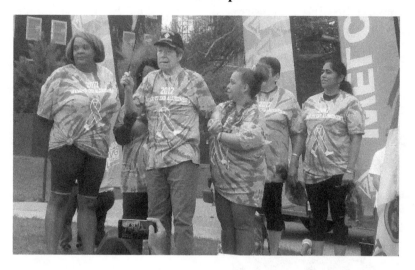

October 8, 2017

POST: *Alzheimer's Walk*

David Finfrock of NBC News was the MC at the Walk to End Alz. Since many of you asked ... I will share what he said of my dad (and thanks for asking FYI):
Please also note that my dad got on the stage BECAUSE of his loving caregivers!

[COL. MARC STEPS FORWARD ON THE STAGE]
David Finfrock:

"The blue flower represents people like Col. Marc and his wife Karen Powe. The Powes have dementia and Alzheimer's disease.

Col. Marc Powe is one of the most highly decorated military intelligence officers in the United States today. Some of his medals include, the Purple Heart, three Bronze Stars, two Silver Stars, the Defense Superior Service Medal, the Legion of Merit, and the very rare Soldier's Medal. His accolades and honors are truly remarkable. It is an honor to have Col. Powe with us today.

As his daughter Alexandra reminds us, Alzheimer's and dementia does not care about your level of education or experience, your upbringing or your strength. Col. Powe is, as his daughters reiterate, one of the greatest hero's this nation has. He fought against terrorism, communism, dictatorships, served two tours in Vietnam and in Iraq, "but could not fight this disease alone." We cannot shrink back in fear or with denial. We must tackle this head on. Walk with us today, in honor of who we once were, in honor of our caregivers and loved ones, and in honor of what our future should be!

If you have a blue flower, please join Col. Marc Powe in raising it and keep it held high."

(there is a sweet irony that during the entire walk, the Col never took his eyes of his blue flower ......)

The backstory to this is when I saw the script that read Col. Marc Powe was to walk up on to the stage, I found Londa from Isle and reported the news. She almost laughed. I asked, "Do you want to walk him up there?"

Her response was instantaneous. "I'm gonna cry." What happened next made us all cry as Jeanette, Londa, Kamal, Christine, and Norma all assisted Daddy on to the stage. They stood proudly (tearfully) with their Colonel. Never did Marc Powe have a greater army of soldiers behind him than on that day.

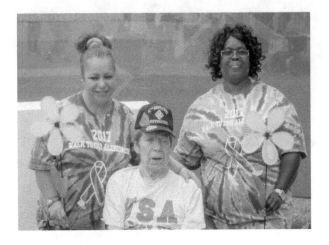

Norma and Jeanette stand with the Colonel

Family, friends and caregivers joined the Walk to End Alzheimer's.

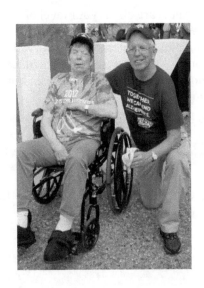

Brothers Marc and Stephen Powe

Additional Resources

American Association of Retired Persons [AARP] – a US-based nonprofit, nonpartisan, social welfare organization with a membership of nearly 38 million, which helps people turn goals and dreams into real possibilities, strengthens communities, and fights for family issues that matter most, including health care, employment and income security, and protection from financial abuse.

601 E. Street NW, Washington, DC 20049

Toll free: 1 (888) 687-2777

Website: www.aarp.org

Administration on Aging [AoA] – an agency within the U.S. Department of Health and Human Services that provides a federal advocacy agency ensuring older persons remain independent contributors of society while keeping focus their concerns as elder Americans. In this role, AoA builds support and uses programs already authorized in the Older Americans Act to heighten awareness among other agencies, organizations, groups, as well as the public, about the value older Americans make to the nation. The AoA also alerts others to the needs of vulnerable older generation. Through information, referral, and outreach efforts at the community level, the Administration on Aging seeks to educate older people and their caregivers about benefits and services available to them.

1 Massachusetts Avenue NW, Washington, DC 20001

Toll free: 1 (800) 677-1116

Website: www.usa.gov

Sample Power of Attorney:

CONTINGENT DURABLE GENERAL POWER OF ATTORNEY

KNOW ALL MEN BY THESE PRESENTS: that, I, _____, an individual residing at _____, have made, constituted and appointed, and by these presents do make, constitute and appoint my [wife, husband, daughter, son, etc.], _____, an individual residing at _____, my true and lawful attorney-in-fact for me in my name, place and stead, to do all things and execute all documents which my said attorney-in-fact deems necessary, advisable or appropriate, in the exercise of the sole, absolute and uncontrolled discretion of such attorney-in-fact, to preserve, protect or promote my person and property, giving and granting to my said attorney-in-fact full power and authority to do and perform all and every act and thing whatsoever necessary, advisable or appropriate to be done in and about all premises, as fully, largely and amply, to all intents and purposes as I might or could do if acting personally.

1.   POWERS – This general power includes, but is not limited to the following specific powers:

1.01   RECEIPTS – To collect and receive any and all sums of money, debts, interest, dividends, annuities and demands whatsoever, as are now or shall hereafter become due, owing, payable or belonging to me, and to take any and all lawful ways and means in my name, or otherwise, for the recovery thereof, and give receipts or other sufficient discharges for the same.

1.02   DEPOSIT ACCOUNTS – To open, deal with and/or close any and all checking accounts, saving accounts, certificates of deposit and similar accounts standing in my name or owned beneficially by me with any bank or other financial institution, including, but not limited to, the power to write checks and other withdrawal orders, deposit funds, transfer funds, and endorse, negotiate or transfer any instrument.

1.03   STOCKS, BONDS, SECURITIES AND DEBTS – To deal with any and all stocks, bonds, securities, debts, stock brokerage accounts, money market accounts and similar property or accounts standing in my name or beneficially owned by me, including, but not limited to, the power to buy, sell, endorse, transfer, exchange, hypothecate and borrow against such property; open, deal with and close accounts with respect to such property. To sign, assign, endorse any stock or security issued by any corporation, bank or other organization and to exercise any rights with respect thereto that I may have.

1.04   REAL ESTATE – To buy, sell, exchange, transfer, convey, lease, re-lease, maintain, raze, improve, renovate, repair, abandon and/or mortgage real property or any interest therein upon such terms and conditions and under such covenants and conditions as my attorney-in-fact shall deem advisable and to execute and deliver deeds, mortgages, deeds of trust and any and all other documents with regard to real estate or any interest therein.

1.05   PERSONAL PROPERTY – To buy, sell, exchange, transfer, convey, lease, re-lease, maintain, improve, repair, abandon, mortgage and/or hypothecate any and all tangible and/or intangible personal property or any interests therein.

1.06   BORROW – To borrow money on my account in any amount, upon any terms and conditions, for any purpose and to pledge, hypothecate, assign and deliver any property or life insurance policy to secure such loan and to execute and deliver any and all documents in connection therewith.

1.07   SAFE DEPOSIT BOX – To open, have access to, and control over and to close any safe deposit box standing in my name or over which I have any control or which contains any property owned by me. To deal with the contents of any such box belonging to me in the same manner as my attorney-in-fact may deal with any other property owned by me.

1.08   BUSINESS – To continue the operation of any business belonging to me or in which I have an interest for any time and in any manner and to terminate and sell or liquidate any such business or the assets thereof at any time and in any manner.

1.09   INSURANCE – To procure, pay for, assign and deal with insurance of any kind and in any amount, and to exercise all rights as owner of any such policy.

1.10   COLLECTION – To take any and all lawful steps to recover, collect, and receive any and all amounts of money or property due and/or owing to me and/or to compromise or abandon any claims or rights I may have and execute and deliver releases or discharges.

1.11   LEGAL ACTIONS – To prosecute, defend, compromise or abandon any and all law suits to which I may be or become a party.

1.12   U.S. TREASURY "FLOWER" BONDS – To purchase for me United States of America Treasury Bonds of the kinds which are redeemable at par in payment of federal estate taxes, to borrow money and obtain credit in my name from any source for such purpose, to make, execute, endorse and deliver promissory notes, bills of exchange, drafts, agreements or other obligations for such bonds and, as security therefore, to pledge, mortgage and assign any stock, bonds, securities, insurance values and other properties, real or personal, in which I may have an interest and to arrange for the safekeeping and custody of any such treasury bonds.

1.13   TAX RETURNS, REQUESTS, CONSENTS, ETC. – To prepare, sign and file federal, state or local, income, gift or other tax returns of any kind, claims for refund, requests for extensions of time, petitions to the tax court or other courts regarding tax matters and any and all other tax related documents, including, without limitation, receipts, offers, waivers, consents (including, but not limited to, consents and agreements under Internal Revenue Code §2032A, or any successor section thereto), powers of attorney, closing agreements; to exercise any elections I may have under federal, state or local tax law; and generally act in my behalf in all tax matters of all kinds and for all periods and for all years before all personal representing the Internal Revenue Service and any other taxing authority, including receipt of confidential information and the posting of bonds and to represent me in all such proceedings.

1.14   JOINT TAX RETURNS, CONSENTS – To join with my spouse or my spouse's estate in filing income or gift tax returns or amended returns for any years and to consent to any gifts made by my spouse as being made one-half by me for gift tax purposes, even though any such action subjects my estate to additional liabilities.

1.15   GIFTS – To make gifts of cash or property, or the income therefrom, in trust or outright, to my spouse, family members, friends and the natural objects of my bounty, including my attorney-in-fact and contributions to charitable organizations in such amounts and upon such terms and conditions as my attorney-in-fact shall deem advisable in the sole, absolute and uncontrolled discretion of my said attorney-in-fact. Any gift by annuity or in Trust may be for a time which extends beyond my actual or expected lifetime.

1.16   CONVEY, RELEASE OR DISCLAIM – To convey, release or disclaim any interest in property, present, contingent or expectant, including marital property rights, and rights of survivorship (incident to joint tenancy with right of survivorship or tenancy by the entirety).

1.17   POWERS OF APPOINTMENT – To exercise or release any powers of appointment, special or general, inter vivos or testamentary.

1.18   GOVERNMENT BENEFITS – To apply for and receive any government, insurance and retirement benefit to which I may be entitled.

1.19 <u>LIFE INSURANCE, ANNUITY, MUTUAL FUND, RETIREMENT AND EMPLOYEE POLICIES, PLANS AND BENEFITS</u> - To exercise any right to elect benefits or payment options, to terminate, to change beneficiaries or ownership, to assign rights, to borrow or receive cash value in return for the surrender of any or all rights under any of the following:

1.191 – Life insurance policies, plans or benefits;

1.192 – Annuity policies, plans or benefits;

1.193 – Mutual fund and other dividend investment plans;

1.194 – Retirement, profit sharing and employee welfare plans and benefits;

1.195 – Employee benefits and employee benefit plans.

1.20 <u>RENUNCIATION AND DISCLAIMER</u> – To exercise any right to renounce or disclaim any interest acquired by testate or intestate succession or by inter vivos transfer, including, exercising or surrendering any right to revoke a revocable trust.

1.21 <u>LENDING</u> – To make loans, secured or unsecured, in such amounts, upon such terms, with or without interest and to such firms, corporations and persons as shall be appropriate, including loans to my attorney-in-fact.

1.22 <u>TRANSACTING BUSINESS</u> – To transact all and every kind of business of whatsoever kind or nature and generally to do and perform all things, and make, execute and acknowledge all contracts, orders, deeds, writings, assurances and instruments which may be necessary, advisable or appropriate to effectuate any manner or thing appertaining or belonging to me and generally to act for me in all matter affecting any business or property which I may now or in the future have with the same force and effect and to all intents and purposes as though I were personally present and acting for myself.

2. <u>DELEGATION AND SUBSTITUTION</u> – My attorney-in-fact shall have full power and authority to delegate any and all of the authority and discretion herein granted and to appoint a substitute attorney or attorney-in-fact and to modify or revoke any such delegation or substitution.

3. <u>RATIFICATION AND CONFIRMATION</u> – All lawful acts done or caused to be done by my attorney-in-fact, or any substitute attorney-in-fact or agent by virtue of this power of attorney are hereby ratified and confirmed.

4. <u>DURABILITY</u> – The authority granted my attorney-in-fact hereby shall not terminate upon my disability.

5. <u>COMMITTEE OR GUARDIAN</u> – In the event it becomes necessary, appropriate or desirable to seek court appointment of a committee or guardian of my person and/or estate it is my wish and desire that my attorney-in-fact herein named be appointed such committee or guardian or in the event said attorney-in-fact is unable or unwilling to so act that a person or persons designated by said attorney-in-fact be so appointed.

6. <u>SUCCESSOR ATTORNEY-IN-FACT</u> – In the event my [husband/wife/son etc.], _____, is unable or unwilling to serve or continue to serve as my attorney-in-fact I do hereby make, constitute and appoint my [daughter/son/cousin/etc.], _____, an individual residing at _____, as my true and lawful attorney-in-fact with full power and authority as herein before granted.

7. <u>CONTINGENCY</u> – The authority of my [wife/husband/etc.], _____, and my [daughter/son/cousin/etc.], _____, as attorney-in-fact to act pursuant to this CONTINGENT DURABLE GENERAL POWER OF ATTORNEY is contingent upon a written determination by a physician then attending me that I am emotionally, physically, or mentally unable or

unwilling to properly attend to my affairs or upon the fact that because of my location or physical status I am unable or unwilling to properly attend to my affairs.

8.   WAIVER OF BOND – It is my wish and desire that no bond be required of any attorney-in-fact acting hereunder or guardian or committee appointed in compliance herewith or if bond be required notwithstanding this direction that no surety be required on such bond.

9.   REVOCATION – I hereby revoke any and all prior powers of attorney made by me and reserve the right to revoke this power of attorney by written document, however, such revocation shall not bind any third party who in good faith and without notice of such revocation acts n reliance on this power of attorney.

10.   INDEMNITY OF THIRD PARTY – I hereby indemnify and hold harmless any third person who in good faith and without notice of revocation acts in reliance on this power of attorney, from any and all cost, loss, expense or liability which arises from such reliance.

11.   LIABILITY OF ATTORNEY-IN-FACT – My attorney-in-fact shall not be liable to me or any of my successors in interest for any action taken or not taken in good faith, but shall be liable only for his own fault, willful misconduct or gross negligence.

12.   PARTIAL INVALIDITY – In the event any provisions of this power of attorney or the application thereof to any person or circumstance shall, to any extent be ruled invalid or unenforceable, the remainder of this power of attorney and the application of such provision to persons or circumstances other than those to which it has been held invalid or unenforceable shall not be affected thereby and each provision of this power of attorney shall be valid and enforceable to the fullest extent permitted by law.

13.   SINGULAR AND PLURAL – Except where the context otherwise requires, the singular includes the plural and the plural includes the singular.

14.   GOVERNING LAW – All questions pertaining to the validity, interpretation and administration of this power of attorney shall be determined in accordance with the laws of [state where you live]

WITNESS the following signature and seal this the ___ day of ____, 20__.

_____

[name of appointee]

[state]

COUNTY OF _____ to wit:

I, the undersigned, a Notary Public in and for the County aforesaid, in the State of _____, do hereby certify that [name of appointee] _____, whose name is signed to the foregoing Contingent Durable General Power of Attorney bearing date on the ___ day of ____, 20__, has acknowledged the same before me in my County aforesaid.

Given under my hand this the ___ day of ____, 20__.

_____

Notary Public

My commission expires:

Thank you for reading our story
and
Good luck with your own travels and trials

…may they be as beautiful as they will be challenging.

CPSIA information can be obtained
at www.ICGtesting.com
Printed in the USA
BVHW07s0918190918
527933BV00024B/1127/P